Doctorate: Finding Your Way as a Healthcare Professional in Research

Doctorate

Finding Your Way as a Healthcare Professional in Research

A practical guide for healthcare professionals, supervisors and those curious about PhD and doctoral studies

JANET DEANE, PhD, MSc, BSc, MCSP

Associate Professor
Rehabilitation Science and Physiotherapy

School of Sports, Exercise and Rehabilitation Sciences
University of Birmingham
Birmingham, United Kingdom

ELSEVIER

ISBN: 978-0-323-87928-6

Content Strategist: Andrae Akeh
Content Project Manager: Fariha Nadeem
Design: Greg Harris
Marketing Manager: Deborah Watkins

Printed in India

Last digit is the print number: 9 8 7 6 5 4 3 2 1

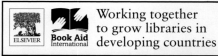

CONTENTS

FOREWORD

This book is an extremely welcome development for a wide range of healthcare professionals who are considering applying for a doctoral course, whether it's a PhD or a professional doctorate, or for those who are already undertaking doctoral studies. To have access to a book that relates to the experiences of a range of healthcare professionals including podiatrists, physiotherapists, occupational therapists, nurses, midwives, speech and language therapists, orthoptists and radiographers will be a huge benefit to all those involved or considering being involved in doctoral studies. The book will also give new insights into the doctoral experience to experienced researchers and doctoral supervisors.

The book consists of two sections. The first section includes 13 chapters based on Dr Janet Deane's personal doctoral experience and journey, including her extensive doctoral process and key learning points. In the section two Janet interviews a range of very experienced healthcare professionals carried out by Dr Deane. The focus of each interview is unique and is very valuable, adding depth and validity to the author's personal reflections. The chapters in both sections provide exceptionally useful and interesting information, which can be drawn upon by those considering doctoral studies, doctoral students and research supervisors in all the health professional fields.

Reading through the book made me reflect on my own doctoral experience. I registered for a PhD in 1981 and at that time I was only the sixth physiotherapist to register for a PhD. Those were early research days for all our professions then! I would have been delighted to have had access to a book like this during my doctoral process.

This book is very accessible to everyone across all the healthcare professions. The range of experiences shared in the book will certainly enhance the reflections of those involved in research and doctoral supervision activities through the encouragement of readers' personal reflections on their previous and/or current research activities. The book also provides a wide range of tips that may help in making decisions and planning the way forward.

The book is an easy read, and those who have a heavy workload don't have to read the whole book at the same time. Choose one chapter that is most relevant to you at the time and read it through. You can pick up other chapters at other times to suit your availability as they become relevant.

The novelty of this book comes from aspects pertaining to the doctoral process that are not always included in other books: for example, being a parent or carer while carrying out your doctorate, career planning, celebrating success, and sharing your experiences for the benefit of the next generation. All of these areas are of great importance for future professional/research activities.

The whole book is an excellent read and, I believe, will be immensely helpful for all those thinking of taking up doctoral studies. Many congratulations Janet on the formulation and completion of this very welcome book. Also, congratulations to all those who were interviewed. I am sure all the information published in this book will be extremely helpful and fulfilling for all its readers.

Ann P. Moore, CBE
PhD, MCSP, Grad Dip Phys, FCSP Cert Ed FMACP, FHEA
Professor Emerita, University of Brighton
Eastbourne, East Sussex, UK

ACKNOWLEDGEMENTS

I would like to express my sincere gratitude to those without whom my research journey would not have been possible. Thank you to the range of scientists, healthcare professionals and researchers who supported my MSc journey at University College London and my PhD experience at Imperial College London and those who continue to support my research career to this day. It really does take a village. Thank you all for walking alongside me and supporting healthcare professionals in research. Trust that I will continue to pay your guidance forward as I continue to support others on the same journey.

A big thank you to the charitable trusts, funding bodies and higher education institutions that have supported my research career so far. To Versus Arthritis for awarding me a doctoral fellowship, to the National Institute for Health Research for my postdoctoral clinical lectureship and to the University of Birmingham for my current position as an Associate Professor in Rehabilitation Science and Physiotherapy, thank you. I would also like to acknowledge those who funded smaller project work, training, dissemination and collaboration, including the Society of Back Pain Research, the United Kingdom Spine Societies Board, Imperial College Trust, the European Society of Biomechanics, the Department of Biology, Medicine and Health at the University of Manchester and the Council of Allied Health Professions Research.

A special thank you to the healthcare professionals who contributed to this book. Thank you for trusting me to share your honest and thoughtful stories. I would also like to acknowledge Poppy, Andrae, Fariha and Vishal from Elsevier for their editorial support and advice. You have understood my various roles, commitments and pressures as a working mum and an Associate Professor in healthcare research and appreciated the flexibility that this requires.

Finally, Mum and Dad, you appreciated my potential when I could not, thank you both for supporting my ambitions. I could not have done this without you. To my husband Hugh and my boys Benjamin and Samuel, you are quite simply the light of my life. Thank you for understanding that sometimes you need to follow your instincts and take courage and time to share your story for the benefit of others.

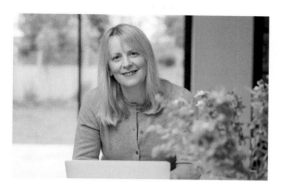

Dr Janet Deane is an Associate Professor in Rehabilitation Science and Physiotherapy and is Deputy Director of the Centre of Precision Rehabilitation for Spinal Pain at the University of Birmingham. In 2015, she was honoured with a Versus Arthritis clinical doctoral fellowship to complete her PhD at Imperial College London. In 2020, she became the first physiotherapist to be appointed as a National Institute of Health Research (NIHR) clinical lecturer at the University of Manchester and Manchester Foundation NHS Trust. The focus of her clinical research is on understanding the mechanisms underpinning chronic spinal pain and facilitating the development of effective exercise, physical activity and digital health interventions for patients.

Janet is keen to enhance research capacity and the capabilities of the next generation of healthcare professionals in research. To this end, she is a clinical academic mentor, supervises master's and doctoral students, plays leading roles in research education and national AHP research strategy delivery, and has developed NHS infrastructure to support healthcare professionals in research. *Doctorate: Finding Your Way as a Healthcare Professional in Research* is the book that Janet wished she could have read before and during her doctorate. This book aims to support healthcare professionals undertaking doctoral studies, their supervisors and those who are simply curious about the doctoral process.

Finding Your Way in Doctoral Research

Real change, enduring change, happens one step at a time.

—RUTH BADER GINSBURG

CHAPTER 1

A Personal Journey

My research journey began when I was a child. Being a curious child, I enjoyed school. On the first day of school my mother packed me off with a little briefcase, to go and learn what I needed to. The briefcase was similar to my dad's and, I suspect, held nothing more than a sandwich. As she waved to me, she was letting me go, preparing me for a future that she would never have the opportunity to experience.

During my time at school, the smell of books and chalk always weighed heavy in the air. In those days it was not always possible to question or to be curious, which was difficult for someone like me. Now as I write this book and share my questions and my curiosity, it is almost impossible for me to believe it. However, as I write, I feel prompted to think more deeply about where and when it all began. When did I undertake my first research project? Was it always written in the stars that a career in research would be my destiny?

First Research Experience

Looking back, there were a few early signs. The earliest sign that I can recall stemmed from an opportunity to undertake a small project at primary school. Each year the head teacher would advertise the project title, and a prize was awarded for the best project: the 'Val Jago memorial trophy'. Although I was a little unsure who Val Jago was, I envisioned him to be a kind man who decided that primary school projects were important. In retrospect, although a simple concept with humble outcomes, it was important. It rewarded curiosity. It encouraged children to have a go at writing their thoughts, a chance to explore their ideas on a topic of interest. As I now know, this project was really my very first thesis.

In preparation for the timely submission of my project, I organised my time well and began to lay out my ideas on an empty page. We didn't have a traditional library in our school, but that didn't bother me. Even at 10 years old, I wanted to learn and was on a mission. First, I just needed to figure out where the books were. I remember entering the little school library that was just off the sports hall. In this little room the shelves were half-filled with donated hardback books, most probably the books that nobody wanted to read. Although it seemed that nobody ever entered or left the room, it was in this little space that I found the peace and time I needed to evaluate the evidence and create my story.

Each day during my break time, I would return to this tiny library to diligently explore the contents. I enjoyed being in my little 'church of books' surrounded by the unmistaken smell of old paper, a smell I still enjoy to this day. Over time, reading from this safe space would become a familiar practice to me. In this space, I was free to explore. There was no right way or wrong way; I was free to find my own way in it. As an associate professor, I now look back with appreciation as I realise just how important these early experiences and opportunities are for young children. Winning the Val Jago memorial trophy as a young child was a seminal experience for me. It encouraged me to think beyond what I thought was possible for myself. It left me feeling: If I could do this, what else could I do?

Who Am I?

As I have advanced as a researcher, I have enjoyed learning from a range of people from different backgrounds, cultures and professions. I find it interesting that no matter who we are and where we come from, in the end, we are all the same. I find it intriguing to learn from experts who understand the importance of knowing who they are and who they are not as they progress in their careers. Experts understand the importance of reflecting on where they have come from to direct where they are going, their values and future careers. Recently I was inspired by one such expert, an amazing interior designer, whose work I have appreciated for its sheer humanity and thoughtful design. As an expert in interior design, she openly shares how her upbringing made her who she is today and how values from her mother and father have permeated her career. It seems to me that in order to move forward, it is useful to look back first.

Writing this book, I have taken the time to reflect on my upbringing and how this has informed my values and research career. My mum was born in a time where girls rarely went to university. However, my mum was a fiercely clever woman, extremely determined and kind. As a child, she moved with her family from place to place but eventually settled where I was born – Cork, Ireland. As the eldest of seven children, she had a lot of responsibility from an early age and took great care of her siblings. My father, on the other hand, also the eldest of his family, was able to attend university. As a trained lawyer, he would later unknowingly teach me to take courage and use evidence to support my case; rather than simply accusing someone of eating the last slice of toast at the breakfast table, it might be a good idea to look at the evidence first. Meanwhile, my mother would teach us empathy; she would consider the personal circumstances that may have led that person to eat that last slice of toast. To this day, it is these values—my dad's courage and my mum's empathy—that infuse everything I do. I expect it is their courage and empathy that underpin why I am writing this book, the book I needed to read during my doctorate.

How to Use This Book

I have written this book alongside my full-time associate professorship, which has been a challenge, but sometimes you simply need to write the book that you needed to read. As a doctoral student, I searched for *the* book that had answers to the questions that I needed to ask, but I could not find it. I needed to understand that I was not alone, that I could be a parent, caregiver and adult learner, and that it would still be possible to succeed.

It would have been easier for me to hide behind the doctoral journey and to make this another scientific publication, telling you what to do based on the best evidence. However, during my doctorate, I did not have the time or will to read any more journals or articles than I needed to. My brain was already operating at capacity, as I expect yours already is. So instead, in Section One, I have chosen to share personal reflections on what I consider to be important doctoral topics. I have chosen to write each chapter, not as a definitive guide, but rather as a point of reference to inspire you to find your own path. I share what worked, what didn't and some tips to get you started. Recognising the importance of personal reflection, each chapter in Section One is followed by space for personal reflection and planning.

In Section Two, I interview healthcare professionals about their personal doctoral experiences. I have taken the time to ensure that this complements and adds depth to my personal reflections. In this section, this highly accomplished multidisciplinary group generously share their honest views on a range of topics. Representing doctoral and postdoctoral students, examiners, supervisors and experienced researchers, they add diverse perspectives that I hope you enjoy.

Overall, I would like you to read this book as I have written it, chapter by chapter. In this way, you can simply read a chapter when you have time, without needing to have read the chapter that preceded or followed it. I have written this for all of you busy healthcare professionals for whom time is such a limited resource. In this book, the style of writing is simple, the chapters short, and there are no references or requirements to do any extra work. It is simply a source of support as and when you need it. If you wonder whether doctoral studies are for you, you are having a difficult doctoral day or you are supervising doctoral students, I hope you enjoy sharing this book and dipping into it to find the support you need.

Finding Your Way: A Personal Journey – Learning Points

- Sometimes you need to reflect on where you have come from to know and understand where you are going. What is your story and where are you going?
- Remember your journey. On reflection, you may appreciate some of the transferrable skills you possess that will serve you well on your doctoral journey.
- Sometimes we don't have role models, but we can become our own and learn from others along the way.
- This book is not a definitive guide, but rather a source of personal reflections to support you in finding your way.
- Each chapter is designed so that the book may be read one chapter at a time, without needing to read the chapter before or after it. In this respect, it represents an easy read for busy healthcare professionals for whom time is a limited resource.
- This book is suitable for those considering a doctorate, doctoral students and supervisors who support doctoral students. On a difficult day, dip into the book to find the support you need.

Finding Your Way: A Personal Journey – Action Points

The most important action points that I can act on today/this week/this month are

Finding Your Way: A Personal Journey – Steps Towards Achieving Action Points

The next steps I can take towards these action points are

CHAPTER 2

The Doctoral Process

It's your road and yours alone, others may walk it with you, but no one can walk it for you.

—Rumi

There is no doubt that undertaking a doctorate has absolutely changed my life. It has given me self-belief, focussed my career trajectory and offered me opportunities that previously I would not have believed were possible. However, I cannot sugarcoat it – it is a challenging road and one to which you need to be wholeheartedly committed. Before embarking on a doctorate, it is important to make sure that this path is right for you. Therefore, understanding the doctoral process from the beginning will help you to set realistic expectations and to make informed decisions for the journey ahead.

Doctoral Whispers

The beginning of my doctoral journey began long before I was awarded funding. Initially it was like a series of coincidences, chance meetings with professors, invitations to present at conferences and to teach at universities. These experiences were accompanied by what I now call 'gentle whispers' that gradually became so loud that I could not ignore them. One of those gentle whispers came from a work colleague on a very busy clinical day. On this day in particular, there was little time for rest. On that day, it felt like people were arriving with painful problems like luggage on a conveyor belt. Waiting times and lists were long, and the system seemed to be bursting at the seams. I remember thinking that there must be a better way.

Having already missed my lunch, I stood there to welcome my next patient. Unknown to me, a junior physiotherapist sat quietly listening intently to the consultation from behind the curtain. Once the consultation was over, I drew back the curtain, and a young voice whispered from behind the curtain, 'I like the way you listen and share the reasons why.' At the time, I didn't feel I always knew the reasons why because the evidence was so limited. However, she was right: I did my best, in my way, to share evidence-based management approaches with my patients. On reflection, this whisper made me aware that I was perhaps thinking differently from other colleagues at the time, that I saw value in evidence-based care, but as the waiting list indicated, we did not seem to have all the answers.

The whispers slowly increased in frequency. Frustrations began to manifest when I would hear clinicians say, 'I manage patients like this because this is the way we have always done it here' or use treatment adjuncts that had little evidence to support their use. Overall, these experiences became a driving force as I became determined not to deliver more of the same. I began to read more, to unpick evidence at journal clubs, to write and contribute to research in small ways. I slowly sought environments in which research was valued and felt excited when speakers would come to share interesting research at our regular in-service training sessions. However, as my confidence grew, I realised that I could no longer sit and watch – I needed to be involved.

Throughout the day, research questions began to fill my head to such an extent that I needed to empty my thoughts onto a page in order to make sense of them. I began to visit research laboratories, attended conferences and spent time with methodologists and healthcare professionals in research. It became my secret obsession. Now, looking back, all of it pointed towards a career in research. It was a slow but gradual realisation and acceptance that yes, perhaps I was different, and that I could no longer accept the status quo. I was curious and felt a personal responsibility to understand and improve the issues that my patients experienced on a daily basis. It was time for a change.

When you become open to the doctoral whispers, they become louder and louder until you simply cannot ignore them. The final nudge was provided by one of my MSc lecturers following my final MSc research presentation. I knew the presentation had gone well but did not realise that I would be awarded first place for my research in my MSc year. Following the presentation of my research, the lecturer quietly pulled me aside and said, 'You have to do something with that talent, Janet.' 'What do you mean?' I replied. 'You need to do something with your research.' This was the moment, the final whisper that I could not ignore. Although I had no clue where to begin, I knew that she was right. In time I realised that in order to progress in research, I needed to undertake a doctorate. Despite all the uncertainties and personal insecurities, when it is your destiny, you find a way.

In this chapter, I present an overview of my experience of the doctoral process from the perspective of undertaking a doctorate in philosophy (PhD). However, as a healthcare professional in research, there may be other options available to you, including a professional doctorate (ProfDoc). Although the structure of a PhD may vary slightly from a professional doctorate (see Section 2, Chapter 2 for further information), there are similar threads that run through both. Therefore, before embarking on doctoral studies, I hope that this chapter will help to demystify the process so that no matter which path you take, you will feel prepared.

What Is a Doctorate?

By definition, a doctorate is essentially a 3- to 4-year apprenticeship in research. The doctoral process is designed to prepare you for life as a researcher, providing the opportunity to learn a plethora of research skills. The overarching aim of the doctorate is to undertake research that makes a significant and unique contribution to the knowledge base, advancing clinical practice and research. The unwritten expectation is that you will be proactive, independent, curious, resilient and reliable, that you will question the status quo, bring new ideas and ultimately make a unique contribution to your research area. However, you will not do this alone. As a doctoral student, you will be supported by an assigned supervisory team, mentors and peers.

Doctoral Assessment

Assessment may vary depending on the university you attend and the type of doctorate you choose to pursue: professional doctorate or doctorate of philosophy. The assessment is usually comprised of two elements: (1) the submission of a written manuscript of your research (thesis) and (2) an oral academic discussion of your thesis (viva voce or viva). Each university determines the criteria that need to be met to pass the doctoral assessment. Since the criteria can vary, it is important to engage with the criteria early on so that you make sure you are hitting the mark. That said, a common theme that tends to underpin a successful outcome is the presentation of quality research that is your own work and that makes a significant and unique contribution to the growing body of evidence in your field.

Following the completion of the doctoral assessment process, it is usual to receive written and verbal feedback on the outcome. On the day of the viva, the examiners, who have been nominated by your university, will have read your thesis in full and will consider whether or not thesis corrections are required. If corrections are required, you will be given time to complete these changes and to resubmit your manuscript. In the rare case that major changes are necessary, a further viva may be required. Once corrections are complete and have been approved by the external examiners, the university will confirm that you have met the requirements for a doctoral award.

Flexible Work

Doctorates may be undertaken on a part-time or full-time basis, and flexible work is usually possible. This means that as a doctoral student in clinical research, you may have the option to continue with your clinical work alongside your doctorate. In terms of doctoral studies, people choose to work in different ways, and there is no best way. For example, I have known some healthcare professionals to agree to a 50:50 split between doctoral research and clinical practice, while some have agreed with their managers to undertake a minimum number of hours of clinical practice to meet their professional requirements. However, I have known others who have chosen to take a career break or to split doctoral life with academic teaching.

Although there is no right or wrong way in terms of how you choose to work, it is a good idea to seek advice from those who have gone before you, if possible. In addition, early consultation with managers, intended research supervisors, funders, family and mentors is key, as this decision could have implications for future job opportunities and family life that you may not have anticipated. However, remember that if one approach does not work, it will usually be possible to renegotiate. In my experience, people care, so if you anticipate a different approach will work better, don't be afraid to ask for what you need in advance. Most employees and funders understand that flexibility will be required, since the doctorate is a lengthy process and your life is likely to change during this period.

Entry Requirements

Before beginning a doctorate, it is important to check the university entry requirements. In the United Kingdom, for example, there is a requirement that students obtain an upper second-class honours undergraduate degree in a related area. Some universities may also require a master's degree. If you meet the university criteria, you may also be required to complete an online application form and, subject to meeting the application requirements, you may be invited for an interview.

Prospective doctoral students are often requested to complete an application form, as universities want to make sure that students have the skills they will require to succeed. The application form is used by academic staff to make a decision as to whether a student is suitable for an interview and is often used to inform the interview process.

As an example, a standard doctoral application form may require you to provide some of the following details:

- *Resume.* The details of the resume layout and content will be specified. However, if this is not the case, a resume (1–2 pages maximum), including your name, brief biography, current position, and employment and education history (including any grants, publications, research-related activities and awards), should suffice. At this stage, don't worry if you do not have any awards, publications or grants. In fact, most universities are acutely aware that sometimes such opportunities are not available to all healthcare professionals in research. In this instance, you could simply choose to share your commitment to research, academic potential and future research aspirations.
- *Research plan.* If you have a specific research idea and know the supervisor that you would like to work with, then it may also be possible to identify this on the application form. If you

do not have a research idea or do not know who to work with, then simply state your general field of interest so that the university may signpost you to an appropriate research team.

Once you have successfully submitted your application to the university and have been accepted into a doctoral programme, you will be notified of your success. If you are funded, through a fellowship programme, for example, it is usual to receive this confirmation from your host institution once your funding is awarded (see Chapter 3 for further details about funding options).

Once formal notification is received, you will be made aware of the terms of your doctorate, including the start date, the completion date and the milestones that you will be expected to achieve as part of the doctoral process.

Doctoral Phases

I like to describe the doctoral process in terms of three phases: the preparatory phase, the doing phase and the wind-up phase. While I accept that this may look different for different projects, I believe it is useful to have a rough idea of these phases before you begin. In the preparatory phase it is normal to feel a little at sea as you prepare for your research. The preparatory phase usually involves finalising your research protocols, writing them up and submitting research plans for ethical approval in preparation for your research. If you are in the position that you have been awarded funding, you will have had to prepare this plan in advance. In this case, the preparatory phase may simply involve actioning the submitted plan and gaining ethical approval.

The doing phase is the most active phase of the doctorate. It is during this phase that all of the data collection and related analysis occur. In this phase, it is common for students to accelerate their writing, publish manuscripts and submit conference abstracts. This phase often provides the springboard from which the final thesis is written.

The wind-up or final phase is largely devoted to writing, submitting your thesis and preparing for your final oral examination, the viva voce. In this phase, having finished your data collection and analysis, you will have the opportunity to completely submerge yourself in writing and viva preparation. If you have established good writing routines and disseminated your research throughout your doctoral journey, you will really enjoy this phase. There is nothing quite like seeing a thesis come together and having the final opportunity to discuss your research at the viva with research experts in your field of interest.

Doctoral Progress Review

During the doctoral journey, students will have the opportunity to review their progress at regular intervals. Each university has specific processes in place to make sure students are on track. In some universities, a progression or transfer process may be required to move from a master's in philosophy (MPhil) to a PhD pathway. In other universities, a yearly review may be required. For example, following the completion of my first year, I was required to submit a first-year milestone progress report or mini-thesis, which detailed my planned research and my progress and future plans. Once this was submitted, I was then invited to present my progress report to two independent academics, simulating the viva voce experience. This valuable yearly experience provided a chance to reflect. It was a chance to discuss what worked and what did not. The detailed feedback I received increased my awareness of what I was doing well and what I could do to further enhance my work. This experience served to enhance my confidence and reassured me that I was on target to achieve my doctoral goals.

Doctoral Support

Universities are keen to support each student through to completion. Here are some examples of the type of support that is usually available to anyone undertaking a doctoral degree:

- **Courses.** There are usually a number of free, in-house courses to choose from when you begin your doctorate. These can range from courses on academic writing to project management. It is important to reflect on where your needs lie and to select the courses that will be most beneficial to you at specific times. However, remember that some courses are mandatory, so prioritise these.

- **Milestone assessments and annual reviews.** As previously described, these processes may vary, but essentially they exist to support you as you learn. Regular reviews can help to focus your attention, to advance your research and to put in place action plans to support you to achieve your goals.

- **Supervision and mentorship.** The doctoral supervisory team will have received supervision training and will be experienced researchers. Although it will be your job to undertake the doctoral project, it will be their job to support you throughout the process to ensure that you are on track to meet reach expected milestones, to offer feedback and to help with problem solving and signposting. In addition, mentorship may be provided by the university or accessed freely through most professional bodies or local or national research networks.

- **Pastoral care and counselling support.** There is no doubt that undertaking a doctorate is a challenging experience. In addition, there are many life changes that you may experience during your doctorate, such as grief or becoming a new parent/caregiver. Free access to pastoral care and counselling is usually available for all doctoral students. Pastoral care and counselling support is provided on a confidential basis, so if you need help, feel encouraged to reach out for the support you require in confidence.

- **Peer support.** At university, there are many societies that you can join. These include sports and cultural societies. If you are changing county, state or country to undertake your doctorate, joining a society may help. In addition, peer support may also be gained from fellow doctoral students within your research environment. In fact, some of my peers have since become great research friends and collaborators. You simply cannot beat the power of a shared experience to bring like-minded people together!

Finding Your Way: The Doctoral Process – Learning Points

- Listen to your doctoral whispers. Be open to the signs that a research career may be for you.
- A doctorate (ProfDoc or PhD) is an apprenticeship in research. The overarching aim of the doctorate is to undertake work that makes a significant and unique contribution towards the advancement of clinical practice and research.
- In preparation for a doctorate, it is important to check university entry requirements.
- Doctorates may be undertaken on a part-time or full-time basis, meaning that it is possible to undertake clinical work alongside your doctorate.
- The doctoral process may be briefly described in terms of three phases: the preparatory phase, the doing phase and the wind-up phase. In the preparatory phase, one finalises research protocols and gains ethical approval. In the doing phase, data collection and analysis are undertaken. The final phase or wind-up is devoted to writing and preparation for final assessments.
- It is usual for doctoral progress to be reviewed at regular intervals. For example, a progression or transfer process may be required to move from a master's in philosophy (MPhil) to a PhD pathway, or a yearly written and oral review may be required.
- The doctoral assessment process usually requires the submission of a manuscript (thesis) and the completion of an oral examination about your thesis (viva voce or viva).
- Following thesis submission and viva completion, written and verbal feedback on the outcome will be given. If thesis corrections are recommended, you will be given time to amend and resubmit. Where major changes are necessary, a further viva may be required.
- Remember that support is available throughout the doctoral process. Support usually includes free courses, annual reviews, supervision and mentorship, pastoral care, counselling, and peer support.

Finding Your Way: The Doctoral Process – Action Points

The most important action points that I can act on today/this week/this month are

Finding Your Way: The Doctoral Process – Steps Towards Achieving Action Points

The next steps I can take towards these action points are

CHAPTER 3

Funding Your Way

The feeling she brought me and my sister up on was: try whatever it is, failure is not the opposite of success but a stepping stone to success.
—Ariana Huffington

Before I committed to a doctorate, I took time to consider the research aims, the project plan, the patient involvement, the provisional project budget, the team and the future impact of my research. However, on reflection, perhaps the most important consideration for me and my family in the end was the financial commitment required to undertake a doctorate. Although it is possible to self-fund doctoral studies, for most, financial support is required. It is a good idea to involve the people who are important in your life in this decision-making process. If they are on board, it will make every financial decision and compromise from then onwards easier. In this way, although you may need to make financial compromises in the short term, it will make it all worth it in the end when you achieve your goal.

Funding Support

In terms of funding support it is a good idea to think outside the box. Academic institutions sometimes offer doctoral opportunities with stipends. However, there are also many funding streams to support healthcare professionals in doctoral research. When you begin to search for funding opportunities it is often difficult to see the wood for the trees. I suggest seeking support from a potential supervisor, mentor, experienced researcher or your professional body to find the stream that is most appropriate for you.

Most research funding bodies have websites that encourage people to get in contact with any funding-related queries. Funders appreciate people getting in touch, as it saves time and makes sure that planned projects are well aligned to intended funding streams. If your application fails to align with the funding stream to which you are applying, you will waste a lot of time and the application will be declined. Since funding bodies have strict criteria to which they adhere, it is a good idea to read the criteria in detail before applying and to check any doubts directly with the funder.

Sometimes funding bodies offer webinars or face-to-face seminars to explain the application process for specific funding calls and fellowships. Seminars or webinars can be particularly useful, as often grant committee members, administrators and successful candidates present their experiences as part of the event. For example, a simple take-home message from one such seminar really changed my perspective on all future funding applications. The message from that seminar highlighted how important it was to 'go in strong': to take the time needed to submit a high-quality application. From this point on, I understood that an application of this magnitude could not simply be cobbled together in a rush; rather, it needed to be a well-considered piece of work in all respects. It was also clear from the seminar that while successful applications take time to prepare, it is important to be tenacious in spirit when you don't succeed.

Different opportunities are offered by different funding bodies. For example, there are personal awards such as fellowships (internships, pre-doctoral, doctoral, post-doctoral), small project grants, bursaries and larger project grants available. In addition to doctoral educational funding, some grants will also fund equipment, conference travel and training packages. Therefore, when applying for a fellowship or bursary, it is important to understand what you can cost for so that you can make the most of your fellowship. Some funders, such as the National Institute of Health Research in the United Kingdom (NIHR), offer a range of fellowships and take a specific interest in training future health care professionals in research. To this end, they fund training that supports the career aspirations of future clinical research leaders. By engaging early with the funder, the funding criteria and related documentation, you will be able to identify the specific funds available, which could maximise the potential impact of your doctoral research.

If you are unsure whether to commit to a doctorate but would like the opportunity to learn more and become more research-active, then it could be possible that applying for a research internship, pre-doctoral programme or MSc in research might help you to decide. Again, funding is available for these programmes. In addition, small bursaries or travel fellowships may enable you to attend conferences, undertake small projects and build collaborations. Research is never a sprint and sometimes you just need to take your time, reminding yourself that each small step you take is in the right direction of travel.

Preparation for a Funding Application

To build a successful application, it is generally important to consider three key elements: the person carrying out the research (i.e. you), the project and the place where you intend carrying out the research. You may have a great project idea, it may be sufficiently novel and represent value for money, but if you do not have sufficient support from a higher education institution to make it happen or if you are not ready to undertake academic research at this level, then it won't work.

The Right Person

Fellowships are personal awards, which some health care professionals apply for in order to begin their doctorates. To be awarded a fellowship requires a lot of personal preparation prior to grant submission. First, before applying it is important to check that you meet the criteria. For example, some fellowships may be open to applications from nurses, midwives, and allied health professions, while some may require the applicant to have a specific number of years of clinical/research experience.

Most doctoral funding fellowships will require applicants to share their resumes, which could include details of education and work experience to date, research experience, evidence of previous academic awards, previous publications or grant awards, transferrable skills (e.g., leadership) and details of the intended career trajectory of the applicant. To ascertain whether you are at the right stage to apply, it is important to engage directly with funders, potential supervisors or applicants who have previously submitted successful fellowship applications to the same funder. Once you understand what the requirements are, you may feel that you are ready to apply. However, if you do not meet the requirements, then perhaps this experience will help you to identify the areas that you need to work on or to consider alternative funding bodies that align more with your needs.

Once you feel you meet the criteria, it is a good idea to engage with the paperwork. Fellowship applications are usually free to download from the associated website or from the funders directly. Most online funding applications can be edited and saved as you go before submission, which makes it easier to add to them and revise them when you have time. By taking the time to review the application form in advance, you will quickly establish what you need to prepare. For example, some fellowship applications support applicants to become future research leaders, requiring individuals to detail bespoke training plans and costings. This can take time to organise since the training plan needs to be focussed, suitably ambitious and worthwhile. Being aware of the application requirements from the outset can really help with planning.

Prior to submission of the fellowship application, it will also be important to engage with local research mentors and/or your respective professional bodies, who will be happy to point you in the right direction for support with your application. For example, in the United Kingdom, the Chartered Society of Physiotherapy offers free mentorship to members, and local research design services can also offer support. In my experience, I have found that if you are brave enough to reach out, most people will be happy to help.

The Right Place

In the early stages of putting a funding application together, it is important to do your research and take your time. Doing it my way meant that I needed to identify the research that I was most passionate about, as well as the best place to carry out that research. Initially, I e-mailed professors with whom I believed I could work and who appeared to have similar research profiles and outputs that aligned with the research I wished to undertake. When I received invitations from these professors to come and meet with them, I took the opportunity to ask about the doctoral processes at their respective universities and also asked about possible projects.

At this point, I must confess, I didn't really know what I was doing. I entered the room as an interviewee with a general idea of what I wanted to do. However, looking back, this was a very weak position to be in. I remember exiting room after room feeling dejected. Sometimes I did not feel inspired by the place, sometimes I did not feel inspired by the research team and sometimes neither. I began to think that perhaps a doctorate was not for me after all.

Weeks went by and finally I came to the conclusion that I needed to touch base with a trusted research mentor and professor with whom I had worked as a research physiotherapist two years prior. As I sat and chatted with my trusted mentor, she made me think twice. Janet, I think the problem is that you are letting them interview you, when you should be interviewing them. Are they inspiring to you?' This reframe turned out to be critical. I suddenly recognised that in my naivety, I had perhaps failed to ask some of the most important questions. Were they inspiring enough for me? Did they have the credentials I needed to support my doctoral journey? Did they have the equipment I needed and staff available to support me? Would they be willing to support a grant application or could they fund my PhD? Would I like to work in this university for the next three to four years? These were important and empowering questions. After all, if I was going to devote the majority of my time to undertaking a doctorate with all of the financial and time commitments this entailed, I needed to be sure that this was a place where I could succeed, where the team were inspiring, where my ambitions and research aligned within a supportive centre of excellence.

From this point onwards, I felt sufficiently equipped to systematically interview a number of universities, feeling assured that eventually I would find the right fit for me and the project. Rather disappointingly, none delivered. This was because, quite simply, I had already found the place I was meant to be and my future doctoral supervisor. Having worked as a research physiotherapist in an amazing laboratory, with internationally recognised and inspiring scientists, it was unlikely that anything else would measure up. However, by interrogating the various alternative options, I finally felt confident in my decision and approached my trusted mentor and professor, who was delighted to support my funding application through her institution.

While this process seems simple, it took years to get to this point and to establish connections. This is crucial to acknowledge, since the decision to undertake a doctorate at an institution is not simply yours to make. Before being able to proceed with a doctoral funding application, it is necessary to get agreement from your potential lead supervisor and the host institution or university. As I had an established relationship with the team and the institution, both the team and I had confidence that we could work well together, and that they had sufficient expertise, facilities and infrastructure to support my doctoral progress and the proposed research.

Choosing the Right Place

Choosing the best host institution is key not only to your future research success but also to your consideration for funding bodies. If funders remain unconvinced that you are in the right place to carry out your doctoral research, then it is unlikely that your research will be funded. Therefore, if an academic centre of excellence is not inspiring to you, does not do work similar to yours and cannot provide the infrastructure that you require to advance in your research career, then it is important to acknowledge this as soon as possible and to search elsewhere.

In choosing the right place, it can be a useful exercise to do some research into academic centres of excellence in your area of research. For example, if cardiothoracic surgery is your research area, then being hosted by an academic institution that specialises in this could increase your likelihood of funding success. Being hosted by a recognised institution not only will give you the assurance that you can achieve what you set out to but also will give funders confidence that the work will be completed to a high standard within a supportive environment; you will be housed within an expert research team with the same interests, and you will have the support you require and access to the facilities you need.

Once you have identified an appropriate academic institution, it is useful to review the profiles of researchers who are undertaking research that aligns with your planned work. In my experience, most professors are only too happy for prospective doctoral students to e-mail them. In this case, I suggest a brief and succinct e-mail that includes the following information:

- Name and where you are currently working
- Research plan (research question and intended project outline). Feel free to attach a one-page project proposal to your e-mail.
- If you don't have a concrete research plan, then provide details of the general area in which you would like to undertake research (e.g., chronic pain and musculoskeletal rehabilitation). If possible, outline the type of research methodology that you would like to use (e.g., qualitative, quantitative, mixed methods).
- Share why it is important to you to work with this professor/university and the impact that a doctorate could have for your future career.
- Include how you intend funding your doctorate (self-funded or would like to apply for funding).
- Finally, attach a one-page resume, including academic qualifications and anything that demonstrates your commitment to a research career (e.g., MSc or BSc research projects, published abstracts/papers, course attendance, committee membership or funding success if applicable).

It is usual for academics to respond to e-mails with a suggestion to meet, or they may refer you to another colleague who may be more suitable. However, some may not have the capacity or may not respond to your e-mails. If this is the case, it is important not to take this personally, to recognise that they may not be able to support you in the best way and to move on. As one professor said to me, and I find it has stood me in good stead to this day, 'if you have the will, you will always find a way'.

Once you have received a positive response from your potential academic host, it is time to consider what you would like to discuss when you meet. Although there are no hard and fast rules here, before you commit to aligning with a specific academic institution, here are a few tips that you may find helpful to consider:

- Supervisor
  When meeting a potential lead supervisor it is important to ask about their expertise. Do they give you a sense that they are as passionate about your research as you are? Have they

published in areas of research that are of interest to you? Perhaps you should consider how many current doctoral students they have currently and how many they have seen through to completion. Could you work with them? What do previous doctoral students say about them?

- Environment

  Does the university have the facilities and equipment that you will need to carry out your research? When you visited the research environment and met with the team, did you feel comfortable? Could you envisage yourself working there for three to four years?

- Support

  Institutions usually provide specific doctoral support, including health and wellbeing services (e.g., counselling services, gym facilities, prayer rooms), courses (e.g., writing workshops, thesis and viva voce preparation) and regular supervisory support meetings. When you look at the website and/or meet with your potential lead supervisor, is this support available?

- Funding applications support

  When applying for doctoral funding, it will be necessary to receive the timely support you require to submit a successful application. Is your potential lead supervisor willing to support you in completing such an application? Have they successfully supported other students to do this?

- Local funding opportunities

  Doctoral funding may be available within the department or academic institution you are wishing to attend. This usually requires a student to undertake a predetermined project and may require an interview. Asking about such opportunities could be a good option if you are unsure about your specific research question or feel that you would be happy working in any area. For example, you may wish to undertake rehabilitation research, so a project that examines rehabilitation in any area could work for you.

- Consider additional costs

  If you intend to apply for funding, you will need to be clear what funders will fund and what they will not. The same is true for projects funded by the university. To successfully complete a doctorate, it will be important to consider the personal costs outside of the project itself that may not be covered by a grant (e.g., accommodation for the duration of your doctorate, travel, subsistence, and other outgoes you may have, including childcare and mortgage). Thorough consideration of your personal budget and requirements to undertake additional work will be important so that flexible working options and financial support opportunities can be discussed in advance.

Project

To successfully complete a doctorate, I believe it is crucial to select an area that has personal resonance. This should be a subject area that you are passionate about, a project that is unique, and for research as a healthcare professional, will have an impact upon the people you serve as a clinician. It is this passion that will shine if applying for grant funding or a doctoral position at any university. More importantly, it is this passion that will get you through the most challenging days of your doctorate and will bolster you as you defend your thesis and disseminate your work. As my father says, doing work that you are passionate about 'makes your good days great and your bad days bearable'.

When I submitted my application for a doctoral fellowship, I had just completed my MSc in advanced musculoskeletal physiotherapy and research and was working as a part-time teaching fellow and clinician. Since I was new to grant writing, I was unaware of the funding bodies that I could apply to for a doctoral fellowship award, so I turned to my intended lead supervisor for support. She suggested a few funding bodies that typically fund the type of research that I was interested in doing. I took the time to go through a selection of websites based on the guidance received and noted the requirements. I also engaged directly with the funders through suggested contacts on their web pages. This process took approximately one month and gave me time to think about the most appropriate course to take. I then presented my thoughts to my intended supervisor and we agreed together on the most suitable path based upon my career objectives (person), my academic host (place), and my doctoral research plan (project).

In terms of the project details that funding bodies could ask you to provide, I have listed a few common themes that arise to help you. Although not exhaustive, and themes may vary depending on the award and funding body, the list below is an example of the details that could be requested. This is not to discourage you, but rather to help you to plan well in advance. Working an application up to a level where it is ready for submission can take 6–12 months or more and requires detailed planning.

List of project details that could be requested by a doctoral funding body:

- Lay summary of your project
- Research question
- Aims and objectives
- Background with evidence to support your research
- Methodology
- Analysis details
- Project management plan
- Dissemination plan
- Potential impact, scalability, and value for money
- How you will involve and engage patients and the public in your research
- Future research
- Details of collaborators, mentors, advisors, co-supervisors, trial sites, and trial management teams who have confirmed their support. You may be required to submit letters of support from each team member, including the trials unit.
- Personal training plan. This is usual for personal fellowship awards.
- Detailed budget with reasoning. Funders may ask you to include costs for patient and public involvement and engagement activities, equipment, facilities, open access publication and so on.

If you are in the early stages and do not have a specific project plan or research question in mind, take some time to reflect upon the literature in your area of interest, attend conferences in related areas to see where the gaps lie, and discuss ideas with your intended team, your patients and trusted research friends. Taking the time and opportunity to question your ideas will help you to develop them into a focussed research project suitable for submission. Be open to sharing your thoughts with your planned supervisor as early as possible. It is important for an idea to fail early rather than for you to struggle on with an idea that is unrealistic and will never come to anything. Through the interrogation of ideas and receipt of feedback from trusted colleagues and patients, you will feel assured that you, the person, the project and the place are worthy of funding.

Be Aware of the Road Blocks

The deadlines for submission of all doctoral funding applications are always clearly stated by funders. In my experience, funders will not accept applications outside of the stated deadlines, irrespective of the reason. Often applications involve a two-stage process. Stage one usually involves a submission of interest outlining the intended work. Once the applications have been reviewed by experts, you may be invited to submit a stage two application. In stage two it is usual to be invited to flesh out ideas in more detail, including details of the project and funding, for example.

In planning an application it is important to work backwards from the deadline in order to plan well and avoid any unnecessary stress. However, despite planning in the best way you know how, you will be surprised how many things can take longer to action or deliver than you had originally anticipated. This is why a discussion with your intended doctoral supervisor at an early stage in the application process and/or a discussion with previously successful candidates or experienced researchers can really help. This will assist you to identify the key roadblocks as early as possible so that you can mitigate them.

During the doctorate there are courses available to you that can improve your grantsmanship for future grant applications. During my doctoral experience I was lucky to be selected through a competitive process to represent my university at a grant writing retreat. It was organised by the National Institute for Health Research in the United Kingdom. As part of this particular retreat, we were required to split into groups and encouraged to develop and submit imaginary grant applications together. This task was designed to engage students with the potential issues that one could encounter in the grant application process. Interestingly, the roadblocks that we were encouraged to think about and experienced in this pretend scenario were similar to those that I experienced in the real world.

With regard to funding applications, being forewarned is being forearmed. Below I share a summary of all of the potential roadblocks that I only became aware of after the fact and would have appreciated advance warning of. You will note that all of the roadblocks relate to time. So simply take the time you need to prepare well.

Remember that it takes time to
- generate a research question and detailed plan that align with the funding criteria
- establish an appropriate team with the required level of expertise
- gain feedback from the team in order to optimise the project proposal
- involve and engage with patients from the beginning of the project and revise the plan in accordance with feedback received
- discuss costings with the university accounting department or additional departments (including any health service involvement, such as the NHS) from the outset and identify any hidden costs in terms of facility use, staff payment and so on
- receive letters of support from your team if this is requested by the funder
- gain signatures from the university head of department, supervisors and accounting department on the final document.

In an effort to set realistic deadlines, consult your intended supervisor with an outline of the dates by which you hope to complete each of the tasks. To this end, people often find it helpful to create a Gantt chart, which they can use to share their plans clearly. This will make sure that you and your team will be aware of when they will be receiving specific information for review or when they need to complete specific tasks (e.g., signing off on your submission, providing comments on a document). In this way there will hopefully be fewer surprises, your team will deliver and you will submit your application on time.

Funding Highs and Lows

If you are successful with your application, you will generally be notified by the funding body within a pre-defined period of time. With personal awards or fellowships, for example, following successful submission and review of your application, there may be an additional interview process before the funds are awarded. When I was notified that my doctoral fellowship application was successful, I was invited to interview by my funder, Versus Arthritis. For a healthcare professional such as me, this was daunting. Although I had presented my research at conferences and had undertaken an MSc degree, I has never experienced a fellowship interview before. As I didn't know of anyone who had been successful in receiving a doctoral fellowship from the same funder, or any funder, in fact, I really didn't know what to expect. However, with the support of my intended doctoral supervisor, I began preparation as soon as I received my invitation to interview.

For the interview I was asked to prepare a PowerPoint presentation. The number of slides, style and headings were specified. The funder also shared the details of each interviewer who would be in attendance and where and when the interview would take place. As I looked through the panel list, I noted that the panel consisted of ten male professors from a range of backgrounds and one female administrative staff member. At the time I was pregnant, so the prospects of such an interview felt a little overwhelming.

On the day of the interview, I left plenty of time to get to the venue. I sent them a copy of the PowerPoint by the required deadline but also arrived with copies saved on my USB drive, in the cloud, and on my computer. I also brought plenty of water and some fruit in case I needed it. My bag was full. I was ready. As I walked into the room, I realised that it was really now or never. As my first experience, I would describe it as a true grilling. I must admit, I felt a little overwhelmed by the number of people in the room, and as I stood for over 30 minutes, I remember the administrator kindly inviting me to take a seat. It felt like almost being in the dock of a courtroom, defending my position.

Unfortunately, two days later, I was notified that I had not succeeded. I was distraught, but funnily enough, being pregnant really helped, as I could not deny that my baby and family were actually the most important thing to me at this time. Although things had not ended in the way I had expected, the feedback indicated that although the project required further refinement, this was the right place in which to do the research and I was the right person for the job. From that moment onwards, I knew my journey was not over. It was only just beginning. With a bit of refinement this project was fundable.

When you fail, and you may, remember that this is just the beginning for you, too. You may not agree with the outcome, but when you take the time to step away from the feedback and reflect, you will probably agree with the decision. In my eyes, the true failure comes when we cannot accept and learn from our failures. Most funders provide detailed feedback so that we can reflect, modify and move forward. The feedback helps us to appreciate that there is something about the project, person or place that is not quite right and that through addressing these aspects we can simply re-submit and go in stronger next time.

If you have failed, it is important to seek advice and further support from mentors, research design services, and your professional body or intended supervisory team. Oftentimes a simple steer in the right direction is all you need to help you move forward. Here are a few tips from my experience that may help you as you find your way when you deal with funding failure:

- Step away from the feedback. Sometimes feedback can be unintentionally cutting or difficult to read, as your project is so personal to you. If this is the case, it may help you to take some time away from it before you begin again. When you return to it, try rephrasing the feedback in your own words so it becomes objective and less personal. Think 'What are they asking me to do?' 'What are they seeking further clarity on?' 'What are the key changes that I need to make here?' The types of changes they expect could be major or minor. It will be important to address all the feedback if you are planning to re-submit to the same funder.

- If you have failed a few times with submitting an application, it may be time to be honest with yourself and to reconsider. Critical friends can be useful at this point. If the feedback you are receiving indicates that there are critical flaws in the science or the project itself, it may be time to reconsider the entire project. However, remember that in research nothing is ever wasted. Keep each version of each application that you ever write; you never know how it may inspire you in the future or how it could be repurposed in the future with amendments.

■ Reach out to others who have had similar experiences so that you don't feel so alone. Remember that all researchers are unsuccessful at some point. It is out of failure that the best stuff often comes. Who knows—the feedback that you receive on one application could make your next even more competitive.

■ Fail early. It is important to receive feedback fast so that you learn promptly whether an idea is working or not. Failing fast means that we can adapt and move forward without wasting time on a project that cannot work and has no chance of being funded. Learning to let go and move on is difficult but can be less painful in the long run.

■ Accept failure as a natural part of your learning curve and as part of your journey towards success. We live. We fail. We learn.

Funding Success

When I initially applied for doctoral funding, I did not realise that it was possible to apply for the same award again. This is important to consider if you have been unsuccessful in the first instance. Now, looking back, I think sometimes it's like my grandmother used to say: "That which is for you, Janet, will never pass you by'. In other words, if it is to be, it will happen. When I first applied for funding I was too naïve, my project needed to be fleshed out a little more, and it was not the right time for me and my family, as I was pregnant with my first baby.

However, with a tenacious spirit and after giving birth to my son, I reflected on the feedback I received from the funder, asked my colleagues and research supervisory team for their advice and began again. I knew I was passionate to undertake the work; I knew it was a good idea; I knew I had what it took. I was determined that I would get there. I followed the same application procedure as before, submitted and was invited to interview, but this time was different. I felt confident I could perform well at interview, I knew I had a good project and had dealt with all of the feedback, and I was going in stronger.

Within two days of the interview, I was on my way to work and decided to grab a coffee. For the first time I decided to sit, drink and enjoy it. As I people watched from the window of the café, I received a phone call from a very excited colleague. 'Congratulations', he said. "What's happening?' I replied. 'You've been awarded the funding. Did you not check your e-mail?' With that I quickly checked my e-mail and there it was, the confirmation that finally I was on my way. I welcomed all of the tears that now drizzled down my face. As people stared, I didn't care, because at this point every tear was a very welcome guest. My family history was changing and I was on my way to becoming Dr Deane.

Grant Expectations

If you are self-funding, the university will expect you to meet specific milestones (see Chapter 2: Doctoral process). When you receive a grant award from a funding body, you will be expected to meet not only the university expectations but also expectations that are more specific to the funder. Funders may require you to submit annual progress reports, to acknowledge their contribution on all related dissemination and intellectual property, and/or to continue to build your network and future research potential as part of your funding conditions. It is important to check with your funder exactly what the terms of your fellowship or grant are so that you can ensure you meet all expectations in a timely manner.

Back to the Future

Once you have received funding, it is easy to forget the journey, how long these applications take and the submission process. To continue on your research journey after your doctorate, take the opportunity to consider future options, projects and plans. People usually begin to do this in the final year of their doctorate, as it can take time for funding to be allocated, which may leave months between submitting your application, receiving notification of the award and the funds reaching the university. Therefore, if you are planning to submit an application for post-doctoral funding following your doctorate, don't leave it to the last minute!

Finding Your Way: Funding – Learning Points

- Undertaking a doctorate is a financial commitment that requires thought and discussion with those close to you, potential supervisors, experts, and mentors.
- There are two funding options: self-funded, where you are responsible for funding your doctorate, and funded, where your doctorate is funded by a research funding body.
- Academic institutions sometimes offer doctoral opportunities with stipends. However, there are also specific funding streams for health care professionals. Seek support from potential supervisors, mentors, experienced researchers, or your professional body to find the funding stream that is most appropriate for you.
- If applying for funding, make sure that your doctoral project is well aligned with your intended funding stream. Stick to the criteria it provides and check any doubts directly with the funder.
- If you are unsure whether to commit to a doctorate but wish to become more research-active, a research internship or MSc in research may help you to decide.
- Personal awards such as fellowships (internships, pre-doctoral, doctoral, post-doctoral), small project grants, bursaries and larger project grants are available. Applications for personal awards usually focus on three important elements: project, place and person.
- In preparation for funding, engage with the paperwork in advance. It takes time to consider the project, establish the team and consider the facilities and equipment you will need and the budget.
- Funding applications often involve a two-stage process: an expression of interest and a final proposal. Applications must be submitted by the stated deadlines.
- If your application is successful, you will be invited for an interview. If you are unsuccessful, take time to reflect on the feedback and seek additional support as needed. Failure can be a necessary step towards success.
- If you are planning to submit an application for post-doctoral funding after you graduate, don't leave it to the last minute. Take time to consider future options in advance.

Finding Your Way: Funding – Action Points

The most important action points that I can act on today/this week/this month are

Finding Your Way: Funding – Steps Towards Achieving the Action Points

The next steps I can take towards these action points are

CHAPTER 4

Project Management

> *The payoff of going through the pain of planning can be huge in terms of increased productivity, decreased stress, and, most of all, intentional alignment with what's most important.*
>
> —Elizabeth Grace Saunders

Project management involves the application of experience, knowledge, skills and processes to ensure that project objectives are achieved on a defined timeline. As part of your doctorate, there are specific project objectives to be achieved. For the most part, these objectives will be set within the first few months of a self-funded doctoral project. Project deliverables will be agreed upon with your supervisory team according to a specific timeline and progress monitored through regular supervision meetings and annual progress reviews throughout the doctoral process.

For funded fellowships, doctoral students will also be expected to deliver project aims and objectives; however, they will do so according to the timeline and budget specified in their funding application. The progress of funded projects is usually monitored using progress reports, which grant holders are required to submit to funders on a regular basis. Progress reports are designed to determine whether grant holders are on track to deliver on time and on budget. Funders may also request additional information regarding the impact of the project so far and future project plans. Progress reports also offer grant holders the opportunity to flag issues that could adversely affect progress so that swift action may be taken to avert or address such issues. As with self-funded projects, the progress of funded fellowships is also monitored by the doctoral supervisory team assigned to the project.

Plan From the Beginning

A doctorate is a substantial piece of work. Effective planning is crucial, as it can determine the success or failure of a project. As a doctoral student, you are expected to be self-directed and capable of managing your own doctoral project(s). Although annual reviews and progress reports will prompt you to consider your project plan and targets, proactively taking charge of your project plans from the beginning will mean less stress in the long run.

At the beginning of any project, I often find it helpful to lay out my ideas on a blank page, so to speak. When considering your research, it is important to think about your overarching research question. To answer this overarching research question, several sub-studies may be required. For this reason, doctoral projects are often broken into distinct work packages. Each work package (WP) has its own research question, aims, objectives and protocol. In research projects, each WP is clearly linked to the next, so that the outcome of one WP informs the following WP. For example, if the first work package (WP1) involves a systematic review determining the effectiveness of a specific intervention, the second work package (WP2) may use the outcome from WP1 to select the intervention used. Work packages are usually constrained by time, in that there is usually a deadline by which each WP needs to be completed; for example, WP1: systematic review (0–6 months), WP2: intervention study (7–19 months).

Through the clear identification of work packages and deadlines, a visual representation of your plan and timeline can be created. Project management systems are available to support this. Software packages can be used to create chronological charts or GANTT charts, or you can simply create your own project management chart using commonly available spreadsheet software. Chronological charts or visual representations of projects are often requested by funding bodies as part of a funding application process. However, for the purposes of doctoral projects in general, a GANTT chart can be used as the basis for project discussions, to enhance team awareness of project deadlines, and can easily be updated as required.

To determine a suitable number of doctoral work packages and realistic time frames, it is important to consult with your supervisory team from the beginning. If your planned project(s) lack depth or breadth or you have too much planned within an unrealistic time frame, it could have a negative impact on your work. Sharing a visual presentation of your plans up front will help your supervisory team to establish whether you plans are realistic, on target and suitable for the doctorate. In summary, when it comes to project planning, organise it, visualise it and share it early!

Break It Down

When beginning a doctorate, it is easy to feel at sea with project management. In fact, it is normal to feel a little out of your depth as you begin. Although you may have set your aims and objectives and have basic project work packages in place, the minutia of project management can be challenging. At this stage, it becomes necessary and extremely useful to break larger work packages into smaller, more manageable goals. A very simple way to do this is to identify SMART goals (specific, measurable, achievable, realistic and timely), which are familiar to most clinicians. By defining SMART goals, you can begin to take ownership of your project/s, pending deliverables and time frames.

Start simple. If you are aware that you need to complete a systematic review within the first six months of your doctorate, then you simply need to break down the steps to help you achieve this work package within this time frame. If you are new to systematic reviews, for example, the first SMART goal could be, 'By the end of this week, I will arrange a meeting with the librarian and my supervisors to discuss the systematic review process and to learn about the expert support available at the university'. Although SMART goals may seem quite simplistic, they can empower you to take action in the right direction. Through the ongoing identification of such goals, you will be able to communicate your intentions clearly, acknowledge your progress and share next steps at supervision meetings, at annual reviews and in progress reports.

When Plans Don't Go to Plan

However, despite your being proactive, working hard, defining goals, visualising plans and being committed to regular progress reviews, sometimes things just don't go according to plan. Therefore, part of your doctoral learning journey will be to learn how to mitigate any potential problems using setback plans. For example, you may become aware that the laboratory you need access to for the purposes of your project may relocate within the next two years. In this case, the setback plan could include (1) setting up an amendment to your ethics to permit research to occur at this location also, (2) identifying staff to support the project at this new site and (3) alerting funders that a relocation is on the horizon and that an extension to the timelines may be required.

While sometimes in research there is merit in being rigid and standing firm with your plans to make sure that your project is delivered on time, in some cases swift identification of problems, mitigation and adaptability are more important. As you begin your doctorate, you may have difficulty predicting issues or solving problems in unfamiliar situations. Although your ability to forecast problems will improve with time, if you are unsure it is best to discuss specific issues or plans with your supervisors in the first instance.

Since a doctorate can take a minimum of 3–4 years to complete, it is inevitable for doctoral students to encounter unpredicted changes over this time that have a negative impact on progress. Staff changes, relocations, delays in ethical approval, issues with recruitment due to changes in patient pathways, equipment failure and escalating costs can all impact your progress. Therefore, it is particularly advisable to consult your supervisors on appropriate contingency plans in advance of submitting a funding application or planning a self-funded project.

Taking Charge

Effective project management requires not only goal identification but also regular evaluation. If goals are not evaluated on a regular basis, you will be amazed how easily a project can run off course. Unlike a structured clinical setting, in which goals and deadlines are clear, within an academic context you will be expected to manage your own project, and define your own goals and deadlines to ensure timely doctoral completion.

A great way to get started is to identify three simple goals that you wish to achieve by the end of each day. If, at the end of the day, you have ticked everything off your list, you will know that you have set a realistic number of achievable goals. With experience, you will begin to note that some goals, such as writing a paper, require more dedicated time than writing an abstract and submitting it to a conference. However, slowly but surely, as you become more aware of the landscape and timelines, you will begin to plan more reasonably and realistically, ring fencing the time you need to complete your project-related goals efficiently in a timely manner.

With experience, you will also learn how important it is to evaluate all delegated project tasks. As you become the project manager of your own doctoral work, there will be times when you need to delegate. From your clinical work, you may be well versed in the delegation process, recognising the need to find someone suitably qualified to carry out the work and the importance of checking in to ensure that the work has been carried out to a sufficient standard. When you are new to research, and you have many projects proceeding at the same time, it is easy to forget about delegated tasks and to make assumptions that all is well. Within the context of doctoral research, you may choose to delegate project tasks to more experienced researchers. However, they may not operate in the same way you do just because they are experienced. Researchers, no matter how experienced, may work at different times of day, produce different standards of work and have different motivators than you. Consequently, before they sign up, it will be important to clearly communicate your request, including objectives and deadlines, and to evaluate the progress of this delegated work regularly. Remember that the outputs will be your responsibility, so it is important to get this right.

However, it is not just delegated tasks that require managing. Members of your supervisory team and project staff will also require management. Don't be surprised if some of your supervisors request that you manage them. As busy researchers, your supervisors and project team will require notice and clear signposting regarding project tasks. Different people work in different ways, so it will be important to identify the way in which the individual team members like to communicate and work to optimise progress.

Don't Sink When You Can Swim

It is easy to feel isolated as you begin to experience mini project failures or make errors in judgement along the way. Always remember that in most cases such 'failures' are largely due to inexperience. In this respect, as a doctoral student, you are definitely not alone. Indeed, it is through trial and error, failure and success that we learn the best lessons in project management. Each failure informs new approaches, and we become more efficient, more adaptable and better able to predict and foresee problems, making us better project managers. It is these transferrable project management skills that we take with us to the next stage, the next work package or post-doctoral project. In this sense, these lessons are never wasted. No matter how unsettling or heavy the failures or errors feel, don't sink, just swim; accept failure as a necessary part of your learning journey.

When you experience failures or make errors in judgement, it is key to share your concerns with your doctoral supervisors, who will be happy to help you. This is particularly important if these concerns have the potential to impact future timelines, costs or the submission of your thesis. Remember that the sooner you can identify a problem, the sooner it may be solved. I can guarantee you that most research concerns can be solved through discussion with an experienced team. An experienced team will most likely have navigated similar if not the same problems in the past, regarding failures along the way as inevitable, so take courage to ask for the help you require.

Share Your Problems With Potential Solutions

During my doctoral project management journey, I experienced success and failure in equal measure. It may comfort you to know that during my PhD, I budgeted for a specific number of imaging scans, only to find that the cost per scan would increase two years after I began the project. Realising that this could impact the power of my funded work, my heart sank. While I could have mitigated this within the grant by costing for predicted price rises, I naively did not. A few sleepless nights later, I carefully reviewed my budget and realised that I had not used as many consumables as I had predicted I would. Therefore, if I could simply gain approval to reallocate a proportion of the consumable budget, the problem could be solved. As soon as I identified the problem and a potential solution, I presented the idea to my supervisor, who reviewed my reasoning and suggested communicating my plan thoughtfully to the funding body at the earliest opportunity. Within one week of my communicating the issue and suggesting a possible way forward, I received approval to reallocate the funds, as they deemed it a reasonable and justified request.

It is for this reason that I always encourage students to present potential solutions alongside any project problems. In this way, it is easier for supervisors to discuss problems, sense check solutions and offer advice when project problems are presented. In addition, funding bodies respond well to timely and clear communication of problems presented in a solution-focussed manner. Funders are aware that not all projects work out the way we anticipate and are keen for projects to succeed. It is most likely that timely communication of any reasonable and sensible project changes and potential solutions will be supported.

Consider Yourself

To ensure that projects are delivered on schedule, it will be important to manage your time effectively. This may mean saying 'No' to things that do not support your project and its progress. Improving your personal productivity may also require carving out time in your diary to undertake specific project-related work, changing environment (e.g., working from home or in the library) or creating boundaries (e.g., using 'out of office' message alerts or requesting study leave from clinical work) to ensure that you have the time you need to focus on specific doctoral projects.

When we think of project planning, it is usual to focus on the doctoral project itself with all of its associated work packages. However, all projects can be impacted at any time by the people who lead or take part in them. For your part, as a doctoral project leader and manager, if you have issues that could impact the completion of doctoral projects, then it is key to discuss your personal needs and requirements in confidence with your supervisory team.

Effective project management requires consideration of your personal requirements alongside the project to ensure timely delivery. As an adult learner, you may have planned paternity/

maternity/caregiver leave, health issues, a change in clinical workload or other requirements that could affect project planning. In addition, annual leave could affect the progress of a project at certain times of the year. Through advance planning and discussion, for example, you may learn that it is possible for projects to continue when you are on leave; it may be possible to delegate some responsibilities for a few weeks or months or for you to work from home to ensure that you are on target to meet your deadlines. If it is not possible to delegate or work from home, it may be reasonable to consider revising the project with your supervisory team so that the same goals are achieved over a tighter or extended time frame. Although the possible solutions seem endless, it is important to note that if the project is funded and changes to the project proposal are required, it will be necessary to request approval from the funding body before proceeding.

Finding Your Way: Project Management – Learning Points

- Project management involves the application of experience, knowledge, skills and processes to ensure that project objectives are achieved on a defined timeline.
- A doctorate is a substantial piece of work, meaning that effective planning is crucial from the beginning.
- It is usual for doctoral project progress to be monitored on a regular basis by the supervisory team and as part of an annual review process. For funded doctoral projects, funders will request regular progress reports.
- As a doctoral student, you will be expected to be self-directed and capable of project managing your doctoral project(s). Annual reviews and progress reports will prompt you to consider your project plan and goals.
- Use SMART goals (specific, measurable, achievable, realistic and timely) to break down larger packages of work into more manageable pieces.
- Project management software packages or spreadsheet software can be used to create chronological or GANTT charts. These charts can support project discussions and enhance awareness of deadlines and are easily revised.
- Since a doctorate can take a minimum of 3–4 years to complete, it is inevitable for doctoral students to encounter change that can negatively affect progress. Mitigate any potential problems by establishing setback plans in advance. If you are unsure how, seek advice from your experienced supervisory team.
- As a doctoral student, it will be your responsibility to notify your supervisors and/or funders if you have any concerns about your project(s) that could impact future timelines or costs or the submission of your thesis. Remember that the sooner you can identify a problem, the sooner it may be solved.
- Intentionally align your plan with what is most important. To ensure timely project delivery, manage your time well and discuss any personal requirements with your supervisory team in confidence.

Finding Your Way: Project Management – Action Points

The most important action points that I can act on today/this week/this month are

Finding Your Way: Project Management – Steps Towards Achieving Action Points

The next steps I can take towards these action points are

_____
_____
_____
_____
_____
_____
_____
_____
_____
_____
_____
_____
_____
_____
_____
_____
_____
_____
_____
_____
_____
_____
_____
_____
_____
_____
_____
_____
_____
_____
_____
_____
_____
_____
_____
_____
_____
_____
_____
_____
_____
_____
_____
_____
_____
_____
_____
_____
_____

CHAPTER 5

Supervision and Mentorship

When you know better you do better.
—Maya Angelou

It is certainly true of the doctoral supervision process that 'when you know better you do better'. At the beginning I thought that doctoral supervision meetings consisted of occasional friendly chats to check how things were going. I had no idea that these supervision sessions would become the platform from which I would begin to develop my voice, establish my point of view, interrogate my values and debate and defend my research findings. However, with time I understood just how crucial this platform was, giving me confidence to share my work with different audiences and defend my approach through well-reasoned argument.

Doctoral supervisors are usually assigned by the university, and their expertise aligns well with your intended work. This may mean, for example, that they have expertise in the methodology you are planning to use or the condition that you are choosing to research. It is possible that you may have two or more supervisors depending on your research, of whom one is usually assigned the role of lead supervisor. If your doctorate results from a successful funding bid, then it is likely that your supervisors will include some of the core applicants on that grant. It is also possible that as your research evolves, you may require additional expertise. If this expertise does not exist within your university, additional external supervision may be sourced by your lead supervisor.

In the first year of the doctorate, supervisory sessions tend to occur more often. However, with time, you will find that the frequency decreases as you become more experienced and an expert in your field of study. During the supervision sessions it is usual to discuss matters relating to your research, such as barriers, successes, project management and recruitment. As I will discuss later, supervision sessions may also be used as a confidential space in which to discuss any personal issues that are impacting your doctoral progress.

Make the Most of It

I learned a lot from my first supervisory session. In this introductory session, we agreed on how often the sessions might be and determined if I required any additional support. Seemingly, this was very straightforward. However, at this point, you are taking on board a lot of information and receiving a lot of training, and there is quite a bit of administration to get your head around, which means that it is often difficult to retain information. In the early stages I would sometimes lose my focus when answering a question and find it difficult to recall information, as my postpartum head was filled with ideas and possibilities. To deal with this, I found it helpful to prepare any questions in advance and to take notes during my supervision sessions. If you find that this is a problem for you in the early stages, remember that this is normal and will improve as your expertise grows.

At the beginning, my weekly supervision was provided by my lead supervisor; however, at times all three of my supervisors were in attendance. This was extremely helpful when it came to discussing results, approving abstracts or publications for submission or planning future work.

Having a multidisciplinary group of experienced research staff on my supervisory team was very beneficial. It required me to be able to communicate in different languages: engineering, healthcare, physiology. It encouraged me to explain my ideas more thoroughly and to become more confident in defending my position. Looking back, each session was pretty much like a relaxed viva voce and they certainly prepared me well for the defence of my thesis.

It is good to remember that your supervision is your personal one-on-one time with your supervisors: It is your chance to ask questions, to discuss your research, debate findings or to seek additional support. Simply put, it can be as you define it. My lead supervisor was entirely flexible, which helped me greatly as an adult learner. However, the approach taken is up for negotiation in terms of the form it takes and the duration and location of meetings, so take ownership of it and mould it in a way that suits both you and the supervisory team.

To get the most out of your supervision, it is sensible to prepare. It is valuable time, which professorial staff do not have much of, so make the most of it. If you value people's time and energy and are professional, you will find that your experience will be more positive. Simple things such as turning up to meetings on time, preparing thoroughly for each meeting, being proactive in terms of organising meetings and requesting support, and giving advance notice of meeting cancellations are some of the hallmarks of professional and considerate behaviour. If you are unclear what the expectations are, it is good to ask for clarity from the beginning in order to optimise your experience.

Keep Your Focus

It is useful to set an agenda for each supervisory meeting. I found it useful to send a focussed agenda to my supervisors in advance. Following each meeting, I would update the agenda to add the action points required to address each item on the agenda. I then forwarded the action points to my supervisors so that they had a record of the meeting, when it occurred and my plan moving forward. If I had misinterpreted any of the future action plans, it was then quite easy for my supervisors to alert me to this. This approach may really help you when you are learning the ropes, and as you enter the more advanced stages, the agenda may be used as an aide-mémoire to track your personal progress.

Supervision session discussions are often inspiring and challenge you to think in new ways. Often ideas are completely turned on their heads. During supervisory discussions, I found it worthwhile to use a notebook to document new ideas and inspirational points of view. Although they might be unknown to me at the time, I would later reflect on these notes and use them as a source of inspiration and focus to shape the latest chapters in my thesis, new experiments and future work. However, as you work in your way, do what suits you best in this regard. If taking notes on your phone or iPad works better or you find you need to ask for permission to record meetings, then do this. It is important to follow your way and to ask for what you need on the journey.

During the early to middle stages of my doctorate, I also found it useful to prepare Power-Point slides to highlight my progress and to share embryonic lab results or advanced graphs. This became a very useful tool; I could repurpose these slides for future presentations or send them to any of the supervisors who could not attend the meeting. However, more importantly, these slides were an extremely useful way to keep everyone on track. For example, during supervision sessions, you may get into heated discussions or be presented with random trains of thought that are not entirely the intended focus of the meeting. Before you know it, you may look at the clock and realise that you only have 15 minutes left to ask the key questions on your original agenda. However, by using slides, it was possible to have my cake and eat it too. By this, I mean that it was possible to have fun exploring different ideas while commanding focus. It is amazing how easily distracted you can become when everyone is energised and offering different solutions to issues. However, your job is to guide the conversation, ensuring that the attention of the entire supervisory team is on the issues that matter most.

Great Expectations

Throughout the supervision process, there is a degree of expectation. Some of it is clear and some left unsaid. In terms of doctoral supervision, the expectations are usually clearly set, documented and available to you upon request. However, it is advisable to be clear about what the expectations are from the beginning so that you have the best experience and outcome. Reflecting upon my experiences both as a supervisee and now as a supervisor, I would like to share several important expectations with you.

It is important to be professional and proactive throughout your doctorate. At the doctoral level, nobody will chase you for documents or to understand why you are missing supervision meetings. It will be up to you. Therefore, it is vital to be self-directed. In this regard, it is important to be able to identify problem areas or barriers and to come up with potential solutions. There is simply no point in attending meetings expecting your supervisors or mentors to provide all of the information you require while you sit as a bystander on your own journey. This is your doctorate, and it will be what you make of it.

Proactivity is important in all aspects of doctoral life. In relation to supervision, it may mean arranging your own meetings in collaboration with your team, establishing a clear agenda for the meeting, distributing this in advance and preparing regular presentations of your work to ensure that you are on the right track. As a doctoral student I often found that if I had a problem that needed solving, it was helpful to identify it and to think about potential ways of solving it that I could then present at supervision sessions for discussion. Through this process, I could confidently present my ideas and solutions and we could interrogate the problem together. For me, this was an entirely satisfying experience. By taking ownership and initiative with your work in this way, you will build your confidence in decision making and problem solving.

If you are having difficulties expressing or discussing issues, you may find that a simple reflective approach helps. As an example, the problem that you are experiencing may relate to poor participant recruitment. In this case, reflecting on what has worked well so far what has not and thinking about what could work better next time may help you to find a suitable solution. This reflection may then be used to facilitate your next supervision session. If we apply this simple reflective approach to the patient recruitment scenario that I have suggested, a simple reflection may look like this:

- *Problem:* poor recruitment
- *What is working well:* ethically approved recruitment via e-mail and poster advertisement
- *What is not working well:* continued recruitment via e-mail and posters alone will not support the achievement of the recruitment target within the agreed-upon time
- *Potential solution:* recruitment through social media, which will require minor amendment of ethics forms, amendment submission and approval of including advertising on named social media platforms
- *What could work better next time:* it will be important to consider social media in future ethics applications

Managing Your Supervision and Your Supervisors

Before I undertook my doctorate, every book I read about a doctorate discussed managing your managers, or in this case, supervisors. This seemed puzzling to me at the time, as I did not understand why I would need to manage people who were clearly more experienced in research and doctoral study than I was. However, the process very definitely requires that you manage all of the aspects of your doctoral work, and this includes your supervision and those who provide it. It is important to respect that like all managers, supervisors undertake roles outside of your doctorate, including their own research, teaching and administrative responsibilities. In other words, although your doctorate is important to them, supervising your doctorate is not their primary role.

Therefore, to get the best out of your supervision, you will learn that it is important to work with your supervisors and to learn more about them and their roles outside of your doctorate so that you may appreciate advanced research roles and the time pressures that they may be under. It is also advisable to understand how they like to work with doctoral students. As individuals, not all supervisors will work in the same way. Therefore, take the time to meet with each of them individually over coffee or in their office or in a way that they suggest. Open communication is the way forward here, so don't be afraid to ask them about their expectations for you and their preferred meeting times and places. Information such as this will help you to plan ahead and to foster a strong supervisorial relationship.

It may seem strange to you to think about it like this, but supervisors, although advanced researchers and experts in their fields, are human beings with work pressures, families and demands. Therefore, sometimes consideration and respect for their needs are also important. For example, some supervisors may appreciate a reminder to meet face to face or confirmation of a deadline by which you would like an abstract reviewed or may value a 'talk and walk' rather than an office meeting at the end of a busy day. In this respect, it is important to meet supervisors where they are, determining how they wish to work while explaining your needs with clarity. This will be your job. Supervisors will not chase you for information or to arrange a meeting. Therefore, you will need to be proactive, recognising when you need help and acting accordingly. While a doctorate comes with great freedom, there is also much responsibility, so embrace this from the beginning to ensure that you have the support you need.

Since becoming a doctoral supervisor, I have truly recognised the importance of meeting people where they are, respecting their time, their roles and their additional commitments. Every supervisor will be different. As a result, you will need to be flexible, as there is no recipe for working with supervisors in the best way. During my doctorate I had three different supervisors, all from different research backgrounds and with different expertise. As you may expect, they all worked differently. There was no right way, but I needed to understand their ways in order to navigate mine. If you have a group of supervisors, there are usually a designated lead supervisor with whom you will meet most of the time and additional supervisors who may join in from time to time. My lead supervisor liked to meet with me once a week in the beginning while I established my protocol. I then arranged ad hoc team meetings as required. As you progress through your doctorate, it is usual for the frequency of supervision meetings to decrease. However, if you have a need for further supervision during intense periods, you may request it as needed.

My lead supervisor worked in a way similar to mine, planning meetings and doctoral commitments in advance. However, others worked slightly differently. All of my supervisors were extremely busy people, and I could appreciate this through my meetings with them. By taking the time to understand how they liked to communicate with their students, the times that worked and how they liked to meet, I gleaned the most from my supervisory sessions. One of my supervisors admitted that he was hard to track down, and often I would need to make sure I was well prepared with clear questions or graphs for his review. I would often talk and walk with him as he travelled from one lecture to another or ask focussed questions as he worked in the laboratory. He would ask me for regular reminders of deadlines and to track him down as needed. Although sometimes this was a challenge, by adapting to and understanding the way in which he needed to work, I benefitted from his invaluable expertise and generous spirit.

Pastoral Care

Although the role of supervisor is generally summarised as an academic one, supervisors also play a key role in supporting students from a pastoral perspective. This means that supervision extends beyond the purely academic realm, so that doctoral students may be supported holistically. As a healthcare professional and doctoral student, you will have a life outside of academia, which could include additional roles and responsibilities. Many healthcare professionals may be undertaking doctoral studies alongside part-time clinical work, and may have parental or caring responsibilities or be returning to academia for the first time in many years, which may impact their doctoral progress if the correct support is not in place.

To this end, supervisors can offer confidential advice to support doctoral students through the challenges they face and may point students to the most appropriate services. Supervisors usually receive training in this regard so that they have the most up-to-date knowledge of the services that are available locally. For example, if you have not been at university for a while and find that you are having difficulty with new software or technology or with academic writing or cannot perform a literature search, supervisors can point you to the most suitable academic skill development service to support your needs. Equally, if you are experiencing financial hardship or require an extension for a piece of coursework, or English is not your first language, supervisors can direct you early so that you receive the support you require without delay.

Doctoral studies may surprise you. I like to refer to them as the Olympics of academia, in that the challenges that you will face and the level that you will be required to work at mean that any chink in your armour will quickly be unveiled when you work at this level. In my case, the chink in my armour that began to affect my progress was that both of my parents were very ill with cancer and Parkinson's and I had a young toddler and baby to support. I was aware that I was feeling low and found it difficult to work. However, by being aware of how I was feeling and how it was affecting my work, I was able to seek support. By sharing these feelings with my supervisor in confidence at an early stage, I was able to get the support I required and limit the impact on my doctoral work. Therefore, awareness of any physical or mental health challenges that are impacting your performance and the confidential communication of these changes with your supervisory team are vital to ensure that you receive the best support. Your supervisors are on your side and will be happy to advise you in confidence so that you have what you need to perform at your best.

However, for some, working at doctoral level may reveal chinks that can be resolved through additional learning support. As most doctoral students are high-functioning, they will have successfully navigated their lives until now by employing different strategies to support their learning. While this works well in most environments, during doctoral studies the same strategies may not be as effective and may need honing. For some students, the first time that they recognise that they have dyslexia or autistic traits is during their doctorate. Again, there is a lot of educational support available for the requirements of individual students, so if you are having problems, it is important to reach out to your supervisors for help so that reasonable adjustments may be put in place to support your learning needs.

Adult Learners

As healthcare professionals, we often enter the doctoral career pathway as adult learners. As adult learners, we have a lot of life and clinical experience to bring to the table. We may have already been research-active clinicians or participated in undergraduate or master's level research projects. At this point in our lives, we largely know who we are, why we are doing a doctorate and where we are going. We are also aware of the sacrifice required to undertake a journey of this magnitude at this point in our lives. However, despite the label of 'adult learner', we still have a lot to learn and deserve adequate supervision and mentorship.

Sometimes, in academia, supervisors and mentors may over- or underestimate our abilities as healthcare professionals in research. Sometimes supervisors do not know what to do with a clinical academic or doctoral healthcare professional, believing that we simply represent more of the same, requiring the same degree of supervision and direction as a student who has come directly from their BSc. In this case, there is underestimation of the translatable skills we possess. On the other hand, it can be that our research skills and capabilities are overestimated, in that it may be perceived that we do not require much help at all. If this is your experience, it will be your job to communicate your needs and your previous experience to your supervisors. As an adult learner and healthcare professional, you do not represent more of the same; you are an individual with many transferrable skills and individual needs. Therefore, to prevent over- or underestimation of your skills and needs, don't be shy. As an adult learner, it is important to be proactive in sharing your experiences, your knowledge and your requirements with your supervisors.

When Supervision Goes Wrong

Supervision is a bit like a marriage. To work well, all parties need to get on. Through personal experience as a doctoral student and supervisor and following discussions with doctoral students, I have learned that there are key characteristics that underpin a great supervisory relationship. Some of the value-based characteristics underpinning great supervision include mutual respect, trust, honesty, integrity and caring. From my experience so far, if one or all of these are missing, it can lead to problems.

Ultimately, it is important to receive effective supervision throughout your doctoral journey so that you are well equipped for the road ahead from both academic and pastoral perspectives. However, when this is not happening, it can impact the entire process and make it a challenge for all concerned. Sometimes the supervisory relationship may not work because you have different personalities or perspectives, all of which may be navigated. However, in general, when it comes to a difference in value-based characteristics, this may be trickier.

If you find yourself in a position where the supervision that you are receiving is affecting your academic performance in a negative way, then it is important to address this. In this regard, open and honest discussion may help. Sometimes discord happens through misunderstanding or things left unsaid, so being open may help to de-escalate the issue. Discussion with trusted friends and family members may also help you to crystallise your thoughts and reflect on whether your concern is realistic and reasonable. However, in the rare case where the relationship is irreparable, it is usually possible to request a change of supervisor. If you are in this position, it is advisable to seek confidential support as soon as possible from the independent adjudicator or ombudsman at your university.

Mentorship

Mentorship is another form of valuable support. Unlike supervision, which is structured and assigned by the university itself, mentorship is usually a more informal type of support. Doctoral mentorship is usually not provided as standard by universities as part of their doctoral programmes. I have mostly gained mentors through proactively reaching out or organically, through chatting at conferences and having shared research interests. In my experience, mentors are people who share their way and, in doing so, help you to find yours, a bit like this book. Perhaps you require a career mentor, a research mentor, a methodology mentor or a lifestyle mentor. Whatever you require, for mentorship to work effectively, it is important to know yourself and to be able to identify the support you need.

For me, mentors have always provided a guiding light in many ways. I have benefitted from career and research advice from mentors who are experienced healthcare professional researchers and from leadership advice from mentors both inside and outside my scope of practice and been inspired by entrepreneurial mentors who have forged a unique path in research. These mentors are people who for some reason I have been drawn to, who have ambitions similar to mine and with whom I have a natural rapport and can be completely myself.

In the past, I have intentionally reached out to those from similar backgrounds, who have caring responsibilities or a career similar trajectory to the one I wished for myself. The 'reaching out' is sometimes the challenging part when you are at the beginning of your doctorate, but you will find that it becomes less awkward as you become more experienced. The process of reaching out is never really discussed and at the beginning feels unnatural. However, in my experience, chatting at conferences or networking at university or through social media is a great way to meet inspiring mentors.

Formal mentorship is also available and, if provided by a professional body, is often free for members. In my case, I was first introduced to the concept of free formal mentorship through an advertisement from my professional body and also through Athena Swan initiatives available at my university. As part of the formal mentorship process, they may ask you to identify why you need mentorship and what you are hoping to achieve from the mentorship experience. This helps to ensure that you are partnered with the most suitable mentor and that your expectations are realistic. Once a suitable mentor is identified and you are both in agreement to move forward, the formal mentorship process begins. This may involve face-to-face or virtual meetings, depending upon mutual preference, and can be held at mutually agreeable times. The outcomes and plans from each meeting are usually documented so that you have an action plan moving forward and time to reflect. During the formal mentorship process, you may request support for a range of reasons: leadership, project management, work–life balance or career, for example. However, it is important to remember that formal mentorship is designed to facilitate you making your own decisions and as such requires reflection and motivation. Mentors will usually ask the right questions and help you to reflect on the process so that in the end you are empowered to make your own decisions.

Peer Support

Outside of formal supervision and mentorship, postgraduate students and colleagues are often a great source of informal peer support. The lab in which I had the pleasure to undertake my doctorate was a diverse community with a range of expertise who shared a common goal. On the hardest days it was nice to be able to share coffee in the communal coffee area or to eat lunch surrounded by people on a similar mission. Often after hours analysing my data, I would recognise the need for a break and would wander into our shared common room. Wordless, the inability to speak now entrenched from hours of data analysis, I would simply sit and listen to stories as hot cups of tea were gently delivered into grateful hands. I did not have to talk; I did not have to move; I could just sit there and they understood. They understood the time and space required to transition from the intensity of data analysis to the normal world of conversation before stepping forward into the next challenge of the day. They understood when a cup of hot tea was the only way forward, when a hug or debrief was required, when it was time to step away from writing a paper or practising a presentation. Their mentorship was sometimes unknowingly given but a necessary breath of fresh air. Although perhaps the simplest form of support, don't underestimate its power!

Rising From the Ashes

At the beginning of your doctorate, you will begin to put your protocol together and feel quite satisfied that all is organised, sorted and seemingly complete. However, what you do not realise at this point is that there is and will be a lot of academic messiness. In supervision or mentorship sessions, there will be a lot of interrogation of ideas, career trajectories unpicked, protocols being ripped up and started from scratch as you see more possibilities and refine your ideas. Your supervision and mentorship will be messy. They will unsettle, as there will often be great debate and heated argument. However, by getting comfortable with the uncomfortable, you learn. In the end it is through the messiness of academic debate and discussion that you arise like a phoenix from the ashes of your former self, that you find your voice and ultimately learn to carve your path in your way. Embrace it all.

Supervisors and Mentors for Life

Supervisors and mentors not only are an important part of your doctoral journey in terms of navigating it but may also play a part in your life well into the future. In fact, almost all of the supervisors and mentors I had during my doctorate are some of my best supporters to this day. They have celebrated my successes and supported me through the most difficult of times. They have seen me grow academically and personally, and now, as I supervise and mentor the next generation of healthcare professionals in research, I try to pay their kindness and generosity forward in the same way. I appreciate the journey. On reflection, I feel that the doctorate delivers much more than a mere qualification. You become an expert on yourself; you learn what you need and how to achieve this and to maintain your sanity with support from your supervisors, mentors and peers. As you travel through the sometimes messy uncertainty of doctoral studies, knowledge comes and experience grows. You know better. You do better.

Finding Your Way: Supervision and Mentorship – Learning Points

- Supervision sessions are designed to support doctoral students. The supervision team consists of experts assigned to you by the university based upon their skills and expertise.
- It is important to share any problems with your supervisory lead or team as soon as possible. Problems may relate to your research, learning or physical or mental health, for example. No matter what the issue, you may discuss it confidentially with your supervisors who will be able to point you to the best support locally.
- It is important to take a proactive role in supervision sessions. The sessions can be as you define them in collaboration with your supervisory team.
- Supervisors are busy people. It is important to value their time and yours. Advance preparation for sessions (agenda setting and action planning), a professional approach (arriving on time, professional communication, meeting agreed deadlines) and being clear about expectations are important from the beginning.
- Manage your supervisors. Get to know them and learn how they like to work. Knowing this from the beginning will help to get the most out of your supervisory experience.
- Communicate your needs and transferrable skills to your supervisors. For an adult learner this will avoid over-/underestimation of the support your require.
- When supervision is not working well, it is important to have an open conversation, or if you are unsure, to check your perspective with a trusted colleague or friend first. In the rare circumstance where the supervisory relationship has broken down completely, you may be assigned another supervisor. In this instance, seek support from an independent adjudicator or ombudsman at your university who will guide you.
- Mentorship is another form of support that may be formal, such as structured mentorship provided by professional bodies, or informal, through engagement with peers who share similar research interests or career trajectories.
- Peer support is mostly an organic type of support that is gained through shared experience. Identify where your doctoral peers gather and join them.
- Investment in supportive relationships is important as you continue on your clinical research path. Remember that the relationship with your supervisors, mentors and peers may continue beyond your doctorate.

Finding Your Way: Supervision and Mentorship – Action Points

The most important action points that I can act on today/this week/this month are

Finding Your Way: Supervision and Mentorship – Steps Towards Achieving the Action Points

The next steps I can take towards these action points are

CHAPTER 6

Personal Development and Career Planning

Leaps get us playing bigger right now.
— Tara Mohr

This chapter is perhaps one of the most important in the book. It is about the continual personal development and growth required both during your doctoral journey and beyond. For healthcare professionals in research, it is possible to feel equipped already in terms of evaluating and planning professional and career-related development. After all, in clinical practice this is a necessary part of our work, ensuring the delivery of the best evidence-based care for our patients and progress in our careers. However, as we begin in doctoral research, the 'why' and the 'how' of personal development in research are not always immediately clear. Therefore, the aim of this chapter is to demystify personal and career development in research through sharing some of the scaffolding that you may require to inspire and support your personal journey.

During the doctoral process it is usual for one's personal development to accelerate. In my case, the acceleration was beyond my expectations, and although it felt exciting, it could also feel daunting at times. As you begin your doctorate, the rate of personal development naturally increases as you become exposed to new ways of working and are surrounded by clinical researchers who challenge the status quo, innovate and think differently. During these times, restricted frameworks that are traditionally used to guide professional development in practice do not appear to be as effective in the research context. For me it seemed as if the old ways of working were no longer serving me in the best way, particularly in an environment where everything was new and expectations were changing. As the goal posts moved, I felt ill equipped. I needed to understand the expectations: what specific development goals I needed to achieve during my doctorate and how I would address them. However, perhaps more importantly, I needed to understand the bigger picture. Why was personal development in research important? Despite inevitable feelings of inadequacy at the beginning, I was comfortably curious and intrigued to learn more. Somehow I felt assured that if I could simply adopt new approaches, learn from others and use some of the transferrable skills I possessed, I could thrive.

Get Out of Your Own Way

As I began the journey of professional development in research, I naturally encountered some barriers. However, I had no idea at the time that the main barrier to setting and achieving my development and career goals was me. In other words, if I were to set doctoral development goals and achieve them, I would first need to get out of my own way. I would need to step up and step into the new me. This would require persistence, resilience and self-belief beyond what I had known to date. Although you do not get to the point of undertaking a doctorate without being ready for a challenge, I knew I would need to take steps forward that sometimes felt uncomfortable. At some points this would feel like stepping into the complete unknown. Although I was not quite familiar with 'how' I was going to achieve this, I felt confident that my 'why', the reason that I was undertaking this research, would carry me through.

Finding Your 'Why'

As clinical researchers we are driven by our 'why' in research. We wish to do the best work to provide better evidence-based care for our patients. Our 'why' in doctoral research is usually driven by patient-centred aims and objectives, without always recognising the personal development required to support these aims and objectives during our doctorates. As we plan for our future careers in research, personal development begins to serve a more specific purpose, requiring us to engage with the specific hallmarks of excellence at each stage of the research career ladder as we look towards becoming future research leaders.

Identifying Gaps

At the beginning, I had no idea what the hallmarks of doctoral or post-doctoral excellence were. However, knowledge of these hallmarks is extremely helpful in identifying personal gaps. For example, through reading the University criteria or hallmarks of doctoral success, I was able to appreciate that a doctoral thesis was an original piece of work, of publishable scientific standard, that required the presentation of a coherent written argument. Understanding that academic writing was a hallmark of doctoral excellence and that it had been some time since I had written in this way, I recognised the importance of improving my writing skills. By enhancing my awareness of the hallmarks of doctoral excellence early in the process, it gave me the opportunity to put realistic writing development goals in place from the beginning.

Converse to Crystallise

Regular conversations with mentors, supervisors and trusted research friends can be incredibly helpful throughout the doctoral process. Through discussions with such research experts, I learned that not only is professional development an expectation in research but also, as with clinical professional development, it is a life-long process peppered with common personal development themes. Although not an exhaustive list, some of the personal development themes most frequently identified by researchers as worthy of development during the doctoral journey include the following:

- Writing
- Research methods
- Data analysis
- Project management
- Networking
- Dissemination
- Collaboration
- Leadership

Of course, this is a personal journey of discovery, and your unique requirements may be entirely different. However, it is interesting that no matter what our area of research interest, we all have learning requirements. As researchers shared their learning needs with me, it encouraged focussed conversations on their goals, their 'why' and how these were changing as they advanced in their research careers. Although your development plan will be specific to you and your 'why' will be different, open conversations with others about development and personal career plans may help to crystallise your personal goals and offer you some inspiration as you navigate your doctorate and consider planning your future career in research.

Career Curiosity

As my doctorate progressed and my curiosity for careers grew, I found it useful to read advertisements for doctoral and post-doctoral careers. I was curious to understand which skills were considered valuable and necessary at each stage. This experience offered some insight into the personal growth required to obtain similar posts, making it possible to create new goals and adjust my bespoke personal development and career plans accordingly. In this respect, liaising with the career development office at your university may also be useful. In fact, were it not for the university pointing me to particular events, I would not have known the requirements and expectations of specific fellowships and would have remained naive to certain career possibilities.

Project, Place and Person

Local and national research events held by funding bodies can be a great way to understand the career landscape as it pertains to gaining future research funding or fellowships. When applying for future fellowships or project grants, it is key to become familiar with the attributes that are prized by specific funders and academic institutions in order to plan your development accordingly. It was through attending such events that I began to understand clinical research career pathways, how funding works and the opportunities available. It also provides a safe space in which to network with similarly minded doctoral and post-doctoral students. Interestingly, it was during these events that I came to realise that it is not only the project and the place (university) that funders are investing in; the person at the heart of the research is also critical. To invest in you, funders need to understand your commitment to research, your achievements and your personal development goals and future career aspirations. They need to be convinced that you will go the distance and that any investment they make will be worthwhile. Understanding this early on can help to direct your focus and support you as you plan your personal development and career goals.

Frameworks

There are many online resources to support researcher development and career planning. Indeed, the Researcher Development Framework is an example of a resource and framework that helped me to understand researcher development more completely. Developed in the United Kingdom, the Researcher Development Framework supports successful personal and career development in research through the identification of key descriptors of excellence (4 domains and 12 subdomains). This framework describes the skills, professional behaviour and personal attributes associated with research excellence at every level of performance. Through identifying where you lie, it is possible to generate your own personal action plan and to evaluate your progress on a continuous basis at each stage of your research studies and future career.

Overall, in my experience, engaging with experts (researchers, funding bodies, career support services) and resources (university criteria, job specifications, frameworks) is critical from the beginning of the doctoral process to understand why development and career planning is necessary. Understanding this 'why' encouraged me to accept new opportunities that I had not previously considered, such as invitations from different universities to present my work, which subsequently led to future collaborations and successful funding bids. In my experience, understanding and engaging with your 'why' throughout the doctoral period inspires the creation and achievement of strategic goals, encouraging focus and the acceptance of aligned opportunities as they arise throughout your doctoral journey.

Finding Your 'How'

Once you understand why you need to focus on specific personal development gaps, it is necessary to focus on how you intend to plan and evaluate your personal development and career goals. However, the 'how' does not come automatically. Indeed, if you do not have a guiding light or role model who has undertaken a similar career path, such as a mentor that you can relate to, it seems perfectly reasonable that you may not know 'how'.

I count myself extremely privileged that there were clinical researchers in my research environment who were kind enough to share their 'how' honestly and generously with me. Indeed, as I move forward in my research career, I feel bound to pay their generosity forward in support of upcoming researchers. However, if you do not have a mentor or a guiding light to show you the way, reaching out to your doctoral supervisors or peers or for mentorship is helpful. In this respect, frameworks may also be useful. As you begin to define the gaps in your development using the Researcher Development Framework, for example, the framework descriptors may provide a useful starting point or springboard for goal planning and career-related discussions (see Resources).

There is no doubt that recommended resources provided by your peers, your professional body, your university department and related funding bodies regarding professional and career planning are useful. However, as I found, you may be surprised by the insight gained from resources outside of your immediate scope of practice. Often when requiring new and fresh inspiration, I found there to be simply nothing better than reaching outside of my own profession entirely. After all, as you begin to self-actualise or become the person you are destined to be, there are so many commonalities between professionals in research. While research questions may differ, the personal development journey is similar. We learn that we have more in common than what divides us. We encounter the same barriers and can learn from each other, optimising our experiences and achieving our goals in new ways.

One of the books outside of my scope of practice that engaged me with how I needed to address some of my barriers to success was recommended to me by a close research friend. It was a book by the author Tara Mohr entitled *Playing Big* (see the *Resources* section). As a child, I was never really encouraged to play big. This was largely because in the culture into which I was born young women were rarely encouraged to play in this way. Now that as I was stepping into new doctoral shoes, I recognised that I did not have the tools to play big or to think bigger for myself. I guess I lacked confidence. One of the reasons that I lacked academic confidence was that I was the first woman in my family to go to university and to undertake a doctorate. Now, looking back at my doctoral success, I can say with complete confidence that this is not a problem. It was not a problem because I chose to let my story be a force for good. The fact that women in my family have not undertaken this level of study meant that I had the opportunity and privilege to change my family history. So, welcome your past in. Let it be the part of your story and the 'why' that drives you forward as you figure out how you are going to achieve your goals.

One of the key themes in Tara Mohr's book that resonated with me the most and helped me to figure out my 'how' was the concept of 'leaping'. A 'leap', as Tara Mohr defines it, is stepping outside of your comfort zone to develop and grow. I have come to learn that for me a 'leap' feels like diving into what I perceive to be a bottomless pond, which I hope has a bottom and in which I will not drown. It's the type of leap of faith that we need to become comfortable with in order to self-actualise and become the researchers we were born to be.

As with any journey, you need to have a rough idea of the destination before you plan how to get there. Before beginning the doctorate, I needed to know the key attributes and skills that Janet needed to obtain to become Dr Janet Deane and why these were important building blocks for the next stage of a career in clinical research. In other words, if I laid my career trajectory out on a table or made a mind map of it, what would this look like?

I could show you the endless maps and plans that I made to support my development from the beginning. However, looking back, I realise that while the plans I made were achievable, they were too achievable. They were small and lacked ambition. As clinicians, we are quite used to setting specific, measurable and achievable goals for our patients. However, I have realised that although such transferrable skills can be used to our advantage, in terms of driving a project forward and ensuring that it is delivered on time, sometimes we need more time in which to create, innovate and consider our personal path.

When I first entered the seemingly nebulous domain of academia, I found it strange. There seemed to be no beginning or end to the number of thoughts I could have, the number of iterations I could perform, the number of experiments I could do. Initially I found this lack of structure frustrating, and so I began creating structure, setting goals at the start of each day to remain on target and creating checklists and writing notes to keep track of my progress. However, interestingly, I noted that non-clinical researchers did not always work in the same way, not working to strict deadlines or in such a constrained manner. While this was seemingly strange, I soon understood that as researchers we need to take time to think and be creative. If we think about amazing innovators such as Steve Jobs, I am quite sure they needed space and time to think about new ideas without constraints. In summary, we may need to be open to new ways of working to achieve our research goals.

Thinking Bigger

To get out of my own way, I needed to think bigger and exit my comfort zone. I needed to surround myself with innovative researchers inside and outside my scope of practice. To do this took time and a degree of courage as I crossed new boundaries with my research, entering domains outside of physiotherapy, including biomechanics, electromyography and computer programming, to learn new techniques to understand the mechanisms underpinning chronic pain in support of more effective and targeted care for patients. As clinicians we need to be brave, to cross the divides, to communicate in new languages and to surround ourselves with people who challenge our beliefs so that we may advance and develop in our unique way.

Schedule It

However, we also need to be strategic. Personal development and career planning take time. It is therefore important to schedule the time you need, to consider what your values are and to reflect on what you would like and need to develop. During this scheduled time, document your reflections, ideas and plans as an aide-mémoire that can help you to track your progress. As part of my doctoral process, I had one review per year, which meant that I needed to submit a progress report to my supervisor alongside suggestions for future personal and career development. Following submission, I was given the opportunity to discuss my plan with my lead supervisor, which greatly enhanced my focus through the evaluation of my goals. However, if annual reviews are not part of the doctoral process at your university, don't worry. It is still possible to document your goals and self-manage your evaluation in a meaningful way. Sharing your goals and plans with a supervisor, trusted mentor or friend at regular, scheduled intervals will make you accountable, empowering and motivating you to keep you on track towards achieving your goals.

Think SMART

Once you have identified your personal interests, your values and gaps in your knowledge or experience, it is important to set goals. SMART goals (Specific, Measurable, Achievable, Relevant and Time-limited) are goals we regularly use in clinical practice; however, they may be used in a research context to focus your personal and career development plan. You may wish to assign a level of priority and a deadline to each of your goals. It may also be useful to consider your goals in terms of whether they are short-, medium- or long-term goals so that the planned completion dates can be assigned realistically.

To achieve your goals, you may need to identify supportive resources, including literature, courses, peers and experts in the area. Identifying experts or people with advanced experience can be key to unlocking many personal development and career goals. By talking with experts, you learn from their experiences what works, what does not and what it takes to be successful in research.

Leaping

If leaping requires stepping outside of your comfort zone in order to develop and grow, then I knew I needed to leap during my doctorate. One example of a simple leap that I needed to take early on in my doctoral journey was to begin to talk with expert researchers at conferences. At the beginning this was a very daunting prospect, as often I did not know anyone and felt entirely inexperienced. However, as a clinician, I should not have underestimated the power of my most valuable transferrable skill, the ability to communicate well with diverse communities. To address my lack of confidence when speaking to research experts, I decided to set myself the goal of talking to three experts at my very first research conference. In advance of the conference, I diligently reviewed the programme and made notes of each of the speakers that I would like to talk with and learn from. However, as is the case with most goals, one needs to be prepared to be flexible and adapt goals according to the ebb and flow of the context. Therefore, recognising how busy these conferences are, I accepted that I might not get to talk to each of my preselected experts. Nonetheless, I remained determined to achieve my goal: I would talk to three people I had not met before and I would learn and grow from the experience. Through taking this leap or reaching this simple short-term goal, I developed connections and grew in confidence. Soon this one brave leap would lead to another. Networking at conferences led to invited talks, presentations and an invitation to become part of a research committee. As my confidence grew, I began to test my new networking approach at conferences outside of my comfort zone, at which my profession was under-represented. Slowly I could feel my confidence building. Soon I knew the language and was no longer scrambling for research terminology to express myself, I understood the expectations; I no longer stood alone. At this point, I could confidently accept my place at the table and enjoy the new opportunities that this one leap afforded me. Remember that one leap almost always leads to another and therefore we need to take courage and simply go for it!

Balance

It is also entirely healthy to take a balanced approach when considering the steps you would like to take towards achieving your development and career goals. Perhaps the new skills you need to develop do not relate to research methods or acquiring more knowledge in analysis. Perhaps, for you, the emphasis is too often weighted more towards academic achievement and you feel that your goals need to be more holistic, reflecting mind, body and spirit. Sometimes choosing holistic goals, such as creative, meditative or physical activities, as part of your plan can feed you more for the journey ahead. Remember that you are the architect of your own journey, so it is important to carve the best path to support you.

One Leap and Then Another?

When we are new to leaping, our leaps are often suboptimal, leading to overleaping or underleaping. I think many people can relate to this experience, and it is true for any student who dares to learn new things. For example, I recall attending a course as an undergraduate about joint pain management using a specific technique. As a novice learner and student, it was no surprise that, following the course, I began to see joint pain in all patients and believed them all to require the specific technique I had learned. I have since observed this to be the case for many undergraduates and newly qualified students. At this point in the learning trajectory, it seems that there is limited flexibility in the system, our blinkered views resulting in overshooting the treatment requirements unless otherwise directed. Clearly there is much to learn.

At the beginning of my doctorate, I recognised similar novice behaviour. I tended to over-shoot the requirements by overleaping and setting too many goals. On reflection, I can appreci-ate how this exhausted my mind and body. However, recognising that it is normal to overleap or underleap as we are finding what works for us, I decided to be kind to myself. It was OK; I was learning. This was an important turning point in my journey. So often, as clinicians, we feel the weight of personal and professional expectations. However, as adult learners, we need to be OK with the messiness of learning. As you learn and grow, you will become more adaptable, less judgemental and more willing to try to test yourself in a realistic way. You will succeed and you will fail, but it's all a necessary part of development as you learn to take your first steps before leaping effectively.

Leap Failure

Sometimes leaps do not turn out as you might wish. Sometimes no matter how much we prepare or how much dedication we apply to achieving our goals, leaps result in failure. I think it is impor-tant to discuss this, as failures are often not shared and can mark some of the most pivotal points in one's personal development, in that failure may result in a new direction, a more refined leap or perhaps a leap that is more aligned with your values. I believe that leap failure is the greatest teacher. If we listen, our failures tell us that something is not quite right or is not for right now. In this way, our leap failures prepare us for our next steps. If we take the time to reflect on failures before leaping again, we can use this time to get ready for different possibilities and new direc-tions. In terms of failure, it is quite natural to require space to reflect on, appraise and reimagine your goals. So take the time you deserve to carefully consider your needs and next steps without apology.

Beyond the Doctorate

On the doctoral journey it is quite typical to think about your career along the way and to make more focussed career-related decisions in the final year of the doctorate. However, life has a habit of getting in the way sometimes, so it will be necessary to be flexible and to plan accordingly.

University career services are a great place to start, as they offer free career advice and support to students. The services they provide can include, for example, interview and curriculum vitae (CV) support, including practice interviews or CV reviews. However, the career services at your university will also be aware of local career advisory training sessions and job opportunities that are available in your area of expertise. Indeed, career services are often approached directly by companies and higher education authorities to share bespoke job opportunities that are not made available on open access platforms. Therefore, through liaising with the career service directly, you may become aware of new opportunities that you had not previously considered. The career team at your university may also hold specific career-related events, which may open your eyes to the sheer wealth of possibilities out there. During my doctorate, I did not quite appreciate these possibilities. By engaging with the careers team, I began to understand more clearly the new and highly transferrable skills I was gaining, which aligned well not only with a career in research but also with jobs in leadership, strategy and higher-level education.

Attributes Uncovered

I engaged with the careers service at my university at the beginning of my final year. Initially I thought it would be a useful way of updating my CV and would help me to prepare for advanced post-doctoral interviews. However, at our first meeting, I realised that the approach was much more comprehensive than I originally anticipated. At the first meeting the careers team invited me to complete several questionnaires. This triggered a process of personal reflection, designed by the university to establish exactly what my personal preferences and values were and which career options would be most suitable for me. It was a chance to interrogate it all and to figure out who I was becoming. The experience challenged me to think outside of the box and provided the opportunity to receive objective feedback within a safe space. However, perhaps most unexpectedly, the team encouraged me to think bigger about who I could become, encouraging me to add to my CV and share more of my attributes and transferrable skills than I was used to sharing. The pre-doctoral Janet would not have appreciated the value of such skills, being more comfortable with hiding these attributes than showing them off. However, on the doctoral path, you begin to realise that there is no longer any reason to hide your skills, your achievements or your education. To progress in your career in research, you need to care less about what other people might think and get comfortable with sharing your achievements, your skills and everything that reflects your academic excellence and future potential to succeed.

Fellowships

The career service and funding and professional bodies are also a great resource when applying for fellowships (see Chapter 3). If you are interested in fellowships or accessing external funding, it will be important to consider this early in your final year, if not before, as funding takes time to apply for and funds are not always immediately accessible upon award. A detailed understanding of the fellowship deadlines and when the funds are allocated will mean that, if you plan in advance and are successful, you will be financially secure and avoid falling off the fellowship cliff.

Post-Doctoral Posts

Post-doctoral positions are advertised on virtual platforms and usually involve specific research projects for which funding is already in place. The project remit is usually tight, and the title, aims and objectives have already been decided on as part of a successful funding bid. Post-doctoral posts are usually not permanent posts, being advertised to be completed within anything from 6 months to 2 years. However, they may offer financial security while you apply for fellowships or consider further research related options.

Following my doctorate, I was offered a 6-month post-doctoral position, which gave me some breathing space after my doctorate so that I could regroup with my family and consider what was best moving forward. It gave me time to thoughtfully consider and successfully apply for my next fellowship. As a parent or caregiver, don't underestimate the benefits that a little space and time following the doctoral journey can give you.

Returning to Clinical Practice

If you are returning to clinical practice following your doctorate, it is important to begin to plan for this during the final year of your doctorate and to set expectations as you are able. Often this is a challenging time for both employers and employees, particularly in working environments where there is no established research culture. You left a clinician and you are now returning to practice as a clinical researcher with a doctorate. This challenge is real.

For some doctoral students, returning to clinical practice seems comparable to returning to your family for Christmas; you have changed, but your parents and family believe you to be the same person, leading to misunderstandings, arguments and tension. However, it does not need to be like this. In some cases all it takes is a little preparation, which could include

- meeting with your team and managers in advance of your return to discuss plans;
- offering to share your research discoveries and their impact at regular team meetings during your doctorate;
- mutually agreeing on new projects that could support service needs while using your expertise;
- considering new job specifications that align more with your new expertise.

It is my experience that, within a supportive research culture, most managers are open to discussing new possibilities and options for your future career that meet the service needs. So it is important to encourage these discussions and to talk openly about your career ambitions and the way in which your skills could benefit practice and enhance research capacity and capability within your team.

Moving On

However, for some doctoral graduates, it is difficult to persist within the same clinical environment in the absence of a supportive research culture. Graduates often share that there is simply no point in undertaking a doctorate and putting in all the effort and dedication to simply return to the same job you had when you left the organisation. For some, returning to the same job is an acceptable compromise, but in my experience, returning to the same position usually leads post-doctoral students to consider alternative job options.

Sometimes changing the clinical environment in which you work is the only way forward. Changing environments can lead to positive experiences for graduates as they shed their old job titles and adopt new roles as experts in clinical research. In fact, some post-doctoral funding bodies actively encourage changing your research environment to support growth and development. However, it is important to choose wisely. For example, moving to a centre of excellence in your area of research expertise may support future research projects moving forward, but it may present a barrier to your research progress if the hospital or university in which you work does not have aligned research priorities.

Finding Your Way: Personal Development and Career Planning – Learning Points

- Professional development in research is a life-long expectation and commitment to excellence in research.
- The 'why' and the 'how' of personal development are not automatically intuitive. Therefore, schedule the time and space you need to understand and design your bespoke developmental plan.
- Get out of your own way. Be brave and identify your development needs early on.
- Take active steps to understand *why* development and career planning are necessary in research:
  1. Become familiar with hallmarks of doctoral success by reading the university doctoral criteria against which you will be graded and frameworks (e.g., the RDF).
  2. Discuss your personal development and career goals with a trusted mentor, research friend or supervisor.
  3. Engage with career support services, read job specifications for relevant future positions and attend relevant events to support your future career development.
- Take active steps to understand *how* you intend to plan and evaluate your personal development and career goals:
  1. Have conversations with your supervisors, research peers and experts.
  2. Use frameworks (e.g., the RDF) and resources to identify knowledge and skill gaps.
  3. Engage with resources outside your own scope of practice and become open to new ways of working or ideas.
  4. Take leaps that encourage you to step out of your comfort zone. Remember that leap failure prepares you to succeed better next time.
- Seek advice from your university career team regarding future career planning, preparation and job opportunities.
- Consider your next steps thoughtfully. Whether you choose to return to practice, undertake a specific post-doctoral post or apply for a fellowship, take your time to consider what will work best for you following your doctorate.

Finding Your Way: Personal Development and Career Planning – Action Points

The most important action points that I can act on today/this week/this month are

Finding Your Way: Personal Development and Career Planning – Steps Towards Achieving Action Points Are

The next steps I can take towards these action points are

CHAPTER 7

Health and Well-Being

All shall be well.
—Julian of Norwich

While it is not within the scope of this book to offer detailed health, well-being or personal medical advice, I feel it is important that we, as healthcare professionals in research, begin to talk openly and share our experiences in this area. Although I do not profess to be an Olympic athlete, or a psychologist, for that matter, I want to take this opportunity to share some of my experiences. I share what worked for me, what didn't and the various challenges I encountered. Everything in this chapter comes from a humble, reflective place. It comes from a place of knowing that I enjoy feeling healthy and well and have learned through the doctoral process that when I don't, it can easily impact my performance. In this chapter, I share some very simple techniques that helped me, with the sole intention of providing a very basic doctoral toolkit of ideas, all of which may be modified or inspire you on your path.

Hold On to Your Scaffolding

During doctoral studies it is common to feel like a reed in the wind, vulnerable and like an imposter in your own life. At the beginning I felt this way because my doctoral foundations were not in place yet. The clinical environment and community from which I came were no longer as easily accessible as before. The currencies seemed to be different within an academic setting; people prioritised different things, had different interests and communicated in different ways. At times it was easy to feel like an outsider, but I soon realised that only I could change this. If I could not speak the language, I needed to learn it. If I did not understand, I needed to build my knowledge base. I slowly acknowledged that it was not the job of others to make this journey easier; it was my job.

It is quite normal to feel vulnerable in the early doctoral phases. Sometimes this vulnerability comes through a basic lack of foundational knowledge and skills, feelings of inadequacy or loneliness as you transition to a setting in which the rules are different and the expectations are high. During this early phase, I often forgot about the simple stuff, such as eating regularly and well or drinking an adequate amount of water. I ignored the alerts of exhaustion and frustration that my body was giving me and prioritised my work. Soon enough I was feeling burned out; I became less creative and found it difficult to concentrate and focus. Being from a family and culture that pushes on despite obstacles can be a benefit. However, increasingly I was finding that my relentless ambition and drive were beginning to hinder my progress. I could no longer ignore the signals my body was giving me. The old ways of working that I had previously employed during my BSc and MSc were no longer serving me well on this marathon. In this moment, I had to admit that I was not caring for myself and that this needed to change.

Early in our healthcare careers, we become aware of Maslow's pyramid of needs, where to self-actualise, it is important to meet our basic physical and psychological requirements. So why is it then so surprising to us that the process of reaching our doctoral potential becomes more difficult when we are failing to meet these needs? When failing to meet my needs, I became physically tired, I forgot things, and it took me longer to write, to come up with new ideas or to problem-solve. For me these alerts were signs that I was reaching burnout. Of course, reaching this point is not ideal, so I needed to find a way to check in with my needs on a regular basis.

During my doctorate, a dear friend introduced me to four simple questions that I could ask myself as part of a daily check-in. Although I can only speak from my personal experience, it was a complete game changer. The four simple questions it turns out, have been used for years in various educational programmes and are: Am I Hungry? Am I Angry? Am I Lonely? Am I Tired? (HALT). Asking yourself these four simple questions can alert you promptly to your needs. If you answer 'Yes' to any of these questions, it signals that it's time to take action. If I was lonely when writing, for example, an action I chose to take was to work in the library or a coffee shop. If I was angry, I walked or went for a run. If I was tired, I often chose to rest by doing a simple meditation or going to bed early. Sometimes it really was a simple as this. Through the identification of your basic needs, you will be surprised how quickly your performance will improve. Once you experience the results, you will never ignore your alerts again; instead you will use this scaffold to realise your potential.

Sometimes It's the Simple Things

Nowadays there are endless ways in which we can choose to attend to our health and well-being. During my doctorate, I realised that curated content on social media suggesting that I start my day with a matcha tea and a reflective diary entry, followed by a 30-minute meditation, green juice and a cross-fit class, was not necessarily for me. Instead, I decided that I could choose something simpler, something that I enjoyed and that aligned with the time I had available.

During the doctoral process it is easy to forget the simple things, the things that made you happy and healthy before beginning your doctorate. If you enjoyed weekly exercise classes, practices or hobbies before your doctorate, you will really benefit from keeping this routine. Although you may need to modify your practices and hobbies due to financial constraints and time, make it work for you by considering alternative ways; opting for virtual options over face to face, choosing to attend a class weekly rather than daily or signing up for free student classes.

Exercise

As healthcare professionals, we understand the benefits of exercise. We know that it needs to be undertaken regularly, part of our routine and something we enjoy. However, why does it all seem to go out the window during challenging times? Somehow when our learning curve is exponential and the pressure to perform academically is high, we seem to dispense with the key scaffolding such as our exercise habits. It feels as if when we are up against it, suddenly we 'don't have the time', 'don't have the money' and most definitely 'don't have the inclination'.

Granted, for some, this will not be the case, and they may find it easier to prioritise and commit to their regular exercise routines. However, for myself, I found it difficult to fit it all in, until I realised I didn't have to. For me, it became increasingly more appealing to mix things up and to consider new ways of exercising that fitted with my schedule. As a busy mum of two with limited disposable income, I chose instead to move and exercise in a way that was efficient and achievable for me: a walk at lunchtime, doing basic stretches at my desk, a weekly swim with a friend, free online yoga classes or talk-and-walk meetings with my supervisors and friends. By exercising your way, you will always feel better. Maybe you will run a marathon, maybe you will go for a walk or maybe you won't make it on time to a yoga class that day because you need to meet a tight deadline. If your exercise plan does not go to schedule, don't feel bad; simply remember that tomorrow's another day.

Flow State Activities

Flow state usually occurs when you are totally immersed in an activity and focussed beyond distraction. During the doctorate, the most common flow state activities are reading and writing. However, alternative flow state activities can also be used to help improve your focus: for example, meditation, playing an instrument or engaging in tasks that give you a sense of achievement such as pottering, the time you take to mindfully engage in tasks including cooking, cleaning your work space or decluttering areas at home.

During the writing phase of doctoral research, the stakes seem high and the pressure to deliver for stakeholders, your supervisors and yourself can overwhelm you to the extent that you cannot think or be creative. It is at these times when you do not have the hours, energy or money to undertake anything too complex that flow state activities such as pottering can really help. I have found pottering to be a powerful tool on several levels. It can help to reduce racing thoughts, it can improve focus, and you always achieve something at the end: the house becomes cleaner, the office decluttered, a nourishing meal is prepared for the family.

Give Yourself a Break!

Holidays provide a chance to reset and connect with the people most important to you. I have always found holidays to bring clarity and inspiration. For a doctoral student it is a good idea to check your annual leave allowance when you begin so that you can plan your holidays in advance. Advance planning will help to motivate you and increase your productivity in the lead-up to your annual leave. I would like to share a few strategies that may help you to get the most out of your holidays:

- Submit your request for annual leave in advance and as advised by your supervisor. Ensure that you have received full approval prior to booking your break.
- Turn on your 'out of office' messenger or equivalent automatic e-mail response. Make it clear that you are out of the office and will not be able to respond to e-mails until your return. Offer alternative contacts for urgent queries.
- Do not be tempted to open work e-mails or messages. If there is a large chance that you will receive an extremely urgent e-mail or message necessitating a response while on holiday, plan a time to check for this communication within strict time limits.
- Share your planned annual leave dates with your team to avoid any unnecessary confusion. Provide a verbal and/or written handover if necessary.

When annual leave seems too far away or you require a little extra, don't forget to plan mini-breaks to refresh and rejuvenate. When you lose concentration or feel demotivated, there is nothing quite like a small walk, a stretch or a run up and down stairs to make you feel a little more energised. Mini-breaks could also include a break from social media, reading your favourite newspaper with a cup of tea, listening to a podcast on your commute home or a 'no responsibility' night off. Whatever your mini-break is, plan it and look forward to it.

Connect With Your Community

Doctoral students can experience isolation during the doctoral process. If you are feeling lonely and isolated, it is important to connect with others, particularly if it is affecting your motivation, creativity and progress. Obviously, connecting with friends and family on a regular basis is extremely grounding, but it can also be helpful to spend time with those who share the same journey. Universities strive to improve student connections in a number of ways, through virtual or face-to-face writing retreats, seminars, lectures and social events. Doctoral research societies and communities also have their part to play during times of isolation by connecting like-minded people navigating similar challenges. If you are experiencing professional isolation because you have transitioned to a new environment or are feeling lonely during the writing phase of your doctorate, remember to reach out and connect. If you cannot find a group that works for you, why not create your own? Don't go it alone.

Talk About It

Through the life cycle of the doctoral marathon, it is usual to experience vast personal change. During my doctorate, my father was diagnosed with cancer, my mother was diagnosed with Parkinson's, I gave birth, we moved house, my husband started his own business, and I experienced close family bereavement when my amazing grandmother died. Although feelings of grief, change, rebirth, growth and death are quite natural, during my doctorate I recall wishing I had the power to simply suspend all of these destabilising forces in order to regain my focus.

As life whirrs on in parallel with the entire doctoral experience and creates new personal challenges, talking to someone you trust can really help. As has been my experience, there is much comfort to be gained from talking to people who are at the same life stage or going through experiences similar to yours. Peers who can relate and appreciate doctoral demands will be your best supporters in the end. Doctoral supervisors will also be very happy for you to raise any issues of concern with them. These issues can include anything that either is affecting or has the potential to affect your performance. Since supervisors are trained by the university to provide both confidential academic and pastoral support, they will be able to help you navigate almost any problem, from financial difficulties and maternity leave to dyslexia. If they do not have the expertise you require, they will be happy to point you to a range of experts including student counsellors, medics, disability services, finance officers or career advisors for free support.

If you have experienced or are experiencing health and well-being challenges, please be assured that you are not the only one. Acknowledging the issue and sharing your story with your supervisor, general medical practitioner, friend or family member can be a great first step. Often, through discussion, you will find answers or solutions such as reasonable adjustments, extensions or a more flexible schedule that may help you to achieve your goals. Whatever the problem, nothing is insurmountable.

Your Blank Page

However, sometimes it is not possible to talk about the things that affect our performance. Sometimes it is too raw or uncomfortable and we simply need time to process it all. To do this, people talk about using reflective diaries. However, to an academic, this can feel like just another thing we should be doing. For me, reflection is more about making sense of my plans and thinking about what might be affecting my progress. More often, it is about checking in with myself in my way.

In this regard, I often say to students, 'get out a blank page' and they laugh. The blank page is my go-to when thoughts are invasive, I lack clarity or I have difficulty prioritising. Your blank page can look however you need it to look; it could be a lined sheet of paper, an artist's pad or a notebook at your bedside. Whatever it looks like, it is your space to write, draw, and establish trends and related actions. On your blank page you can make sense of it all in your way so that when doctoral thoughts invade your sleep, you can take the ideas from your head, secure them on a page and rest easy.

Step Away From Your Energy Drains

A doctorate is very much a time for self-reflection. It is a time to manage your energy and to consider what drains it and what replenishes it. As healthcare professionals we are active listeners, care about people and are good at problem solving, which affects our relationships with people and can affect our energy levels during doctoral studies. Simple things such as surrounding yourself with those who nourish and energise you can help. Similarly, putting boundaries in place for those who drain your energy becomes essential: setting clear and limited meeting times or editing friends who no longer support you in the way you need to be supported. In this sense, you will become your own energy gatekeeper. You get to choose who and what you give your energy to, so choose wisely.

Social media can be another secret stealer of energy if not managed well. Although a seemingly innocent source of community, connection and inspiration, if you do not have boundaries in place, it could impact you. In this age, when there is a need to keep on top of upcoming research and innovation, to maintain connection and to build new collaborations, while building research capacity and capability, I have found that social media can help, if used wisely.

At the beginning of my doctorate, I was a total social media novice. As a novice, social media can lure you to share information in ways that may not feel natural to you or encourage you to compare yourself with others. In this way social media have the potential to squander your time, affect your core values and make you feel inadequate. For these reasons, it is necessary to manage social media in your way, to be aware of how they make you feel and to try different ways of working with them. Through experimentation, I have found it most helpful to schedule specific days and times to scroll and post content each week. I choose to share deliberately, with purpose and in accordance with my values. I choose to follow people who share similar values and block those who do not. Perhaps most importantly, I take breaks on annual leave days and weekends. In this way, I manage my energy in a way that feels comfortable to me.

When It's Time to Go Home

Home, wherever that is for you, is the place you go when you need space and time. For me, home represents the space where I can take a breath, where being me is enough and where love and comfort reside. At the beginning of my doctorate, I did not understand the importance of having a place where I could lay my head and forget about the world for a while. Instead, I worked conscientiously without breaks, thinking that by working harder I could achieve more. What I did not appreciate from the beginning is that a doctorate will quite happily take all that you have to give. A doctorate will take every minute, hour and day that you are willing to put into it, without apology. Unless you create boundaries there will be no fun, no family, no hobbies. There will be no balance.

One September day at the beginning of my PhD experience, I began my day as I usually did: got the kids ready for nursery, grabbed a quick coffee, kissed my husband as if he were a passing train and ran out the door. I ran to the bus, ran along the river to make it on time for my first research participant, dropped my bags at my desk and assembled all of the relevant laboratory equipment needed for the day, and as the first participant entered the room, I felt as if I had already completed a day's work. Then I was off to the MRI department, up to the lab to complete experiments, no time for lunch, a quick cup of tea and then on to the next participant. Honestly, it sometimes felt as if I were a passenger in my own life, running everywhere, racing in a rhythmic routine.

However, that day would mark the beginning of the end of that way of working. At the end of this particular day, I recall how exhausted I felt. I had no more to give. As I began to clear up and plan which route I would take back to the nursery to avoid the London traffic, my lead supervisor entered the laboratory and said, knowingly, five simple words: 'It's time to go home.' Just when it felt as if I could not give myself permission to do this, she gave me the permission I needed. It was clear to me that, through experience, she knew when to call it a day. As an experienced researcher, she knew the signs and understood that sometimes there is only one way to go. You need to go home.

In giving me the permission that I could not give myself, my supervisor freed me from the punishing schedule that I had created and made me realise that I could not go on in this way. It was not sustainable. To this day my supervisor does not know how important this was to me. By saying, 'Go home,' she gave me permission to go home to my family, to get perspective, to reflect and make the appropriate changes. In this moment I realised that I was expending all of my energy on my work, leaving myself with little energy for the people who were most important in my life. I knew that I could not continue in this way and so I began to create boundaries to be the mum, wife and caregiver that I needed to.

Boundaries will look different for everyone. It will be important to revisit your boundaries regularly, as things will change with time. I often find that most students know what they need and I hope that through sharing some of my ideas you will be inspired to think about some of your boundaries. Here are some simple boundaries that I put in place to ensure that I could 'go home' each day:

- Treat every day like a workday (9–5 pm).
- Use the final 30 minutes of your workday to prepare for the following day.
- Feel more comfortable in sharing the reasons that you need to leave work on time.
- When your day is done, your day is done. Take time to relax and enjoy the rest of it.
- When your day is complete, say 'no' to anything that cannot be left until the following day.

Working From Home

As academic work life changes, it is becoming more acceptable to work from home and to work flexible hours. Working from home as a doctoral student comes with its own challenges. At home it's amazing how minutes of writing alone or days without exercise turns into hours or months. In time, this can impact your health and well-being. If you find that working from home is having a negative impact, here are a few tips that I have found helpful:

- Set a strict beginning and end to your day. Avoid working outside of these hours.
- Schedule time for lunch and exercise throughout your working week.
- Ritualise your working day. Routine really helps, so when working from home, at roughly the same time each morning, I start my day with a 20-minute 'walk to work', make a cup of coffee, clean my desk and begin to write. Through association, my brain then knows it's time to begin work.
- Dress for the occasion. It's amazing how getting dressed for work can help your performance.
- Virtual meetings can easily run from one to the next, leaving little time to transition. It is important to ensure that you schedule time for a five or ten minute break between meetings.
- At the end of a working day, try to take some time before engaging with anyone. In the absence of a commute, pencil in some transition time to help you wind down. This could include listening to some nice music, preparing for dinner with noise reduction headphones, listening to a podcast, going for a walk or whatever works for you.

Be the Change You Wish to See

As doctoral students and beyond, I think it is important that we become the change we wish to see in a culture where hard work and punishing schedules are often celebrated. Although I feel the tides are turning and awareness is increasing, we have to accept that there is a way to go. For this reason, never forget to share your health and well-being stories, resources or nuggets of wisdom to help a colleague or student experiencing difficulties. Be the friend to others that you needed when you were at the same stage and continue to share this wisdom beyond your doctoral journey.

All Shall Be Well

It is difficult to think that 'all shall be well' when you begin a doctorate, because in simple terms, how can anyone assure you that it will be? When I was young and worried about trying something new, I remember my mother and grandmothers would say, 'It'll all work out in the end.' Sometimes this is difficult to hear, because how does anyone know? However, with experience, I have learned that you will support your health and well-being in the best way by knowing what you need on your doctoral journey and doing that. All shall be well because it will be your health and well-being journey and you will navigate it your way.

Finding Your Way: Health and Well-Being – Learning Points

- It is not within the scope of this book to offer detailed health, well-being or personal medical advice. However, this chapter provides a very basic doctoral toolkit of ideas based upon my personal experience, all of which may be modified or inspire you on your path.
- As a doctoral student, it will be your job to acknowledge and share your health and well-being needs. If you have experienced or are experiencing health and well-being challenges, please be assured that you are not the only one. Acknowledging the issue and sharing your story with your supervisor, general medical practitioner, friend or family member can be a great first step.
- Don't ignore your health and well-being alerts. Use the following questions regularly to alert you to address your needs: Am I Hungry? Am I Angry? Am I Lonely? Am I Tired? (HALT).
- Don't forget the practices, hobbies and exercise rituals that made you happy and healthy before beginning your doctorate. If you enjoyed weekly exercise classes, practices or hobbies before your doctorate, then try to keep this routine and modify as needed.
- Consider managing your energy, flow state and 'blank page' activities to help reduce racing thoughts, improve focus and give you a sense of accomplishment on difficult doctoral days.
- Check your annual leave allowance. Plan your holidays in advance to help motivate you and increase your productivity. Don't forget that mini-breaks in your day are also a great way to refresh and rejuvenate.
- If you are feeling lonely and isolated, it is important to connect with others, particularly if it is affecting your motivation, creativity and progress. Connecting with friends and family on a regular basis, attending doctoral events hosted by the university or joining a doctoral research communities or societies could really help.
- Be the change you wish to see. Be the friend to others that you needed when you were at the same stage and continue to share this wisdom beyond your doctoral journey.

Finding Your Way: Health and Well-Being – Action Points

The most important action points that I can act on today/this week/this month are

Finding Your Way: Health and Well-Being – Steps Towards Achieving the Action Points

The next steps I can take towards these action points are

_____
_____
_____
_____
_____
_____
_____
_____
_____
_____
_____
_____
_____
_____
_____
_____
_____
_____
_____
_____
_____
_____
_____
_____
_____
_____
_____
_____
_____
_____
_____
_____
_____
_____
_____
_____
_____
_____
_____
_____
_____
_____
_____
_____
_____
_____
_____
_____
_____
_____
_____

CHAPTER 8

The Doctoral Parent and Caregiver

To be a good parent you need to take care of yourself so that you can have the physical and emotional energy to take care of your family.

—Michelle Obama

In research it is common to learn from the academic experiences of others and in return to share your experience and 'pass it on'. However, I did not anticipate just how important it would be to learn from the personal experiences of fellow academic parents and caregivers during my doctorate. When I applied for doctoral funding, I had no idea that within the very same year I would become pregnant with my first child. This was largely because, after years of failed fertility treatment, I resigned myself to the fact that perhaps my being a mum was not to be. While this came with great sadness, this experience encouraged me to make the very best of whatever opportunities came my way. It was a turning point. From then on, I knew I needed to have a career that not only was challenging but also could have impact for others.

However, like all good things in life, you can never quite predict or plan what's going to happen next, and so almost like buses that are delayed and then suddenly arrive at your stop together, I became pregnant and my doctoral funding was awarded. Although the timing seemed less than ideal, with the support of my husband and family I decided that this opportunity was hard fought for and that I needed to embrace it. At the time I had no idea how it would all work out, and so faith played a large part in steering me forward. Sometimes you know something feels right but you don't always know why or how you are going to get there. Sometimes it is just about instinct and having good people around you to sense check and support your choices.

By the time I began my doctorate, my son was 1 year old. This helped, because we had some sort of routine at this point and felt more confident as parents. However, I use the word 'routine' loosely because, as any parent of or caregiver for young children will know, such a routine can fall apart at any time without warning. For me, this unpredictability was extremely difficult at the beginning. The experiences and hurdles I would need to navigate were largely out of my control.

That said, it is important to remember that there is a lot that is under your control and that there is support available if you look for it. In my case, there was no chance of direct family support with childcare, as my parents and in-laws lived too far away. However, there were many childcare facilities near our apartment and within the university itself. This led to many an agonising hour, considering which childcare option would suit us best. This decision also came with a tremendous feeling of guilt, in knowing that I was not going to be a traditional 'stay at home' parent and that this could somehow affect my children and their future.

However, I can now speak from experience and tell you that being a working parent did not affect my children in any appreciable way. In fact, I feel that my children had more time with me than I did with my own parents because of the way my husband and I structured our time. Did they miss me sometimes when I was at a conference or working late? Yes. Did they want me to be there in person to feed and clothe them every day? Yes. In fact, who wouldn't? However, I believe there is a balance that can be struck that benefits all.

For a doctoral student it is normal to experiences certain pressures on given days, weeks or months. There will be deadlines that need to be met during your doctorate, and the expectations are high. However, do not let this overwhelm you. Instead, consider the possibility that the experience can be a positive one. Although, in the end, the doctoral parent or caregiver journey will be entirely as you define it, I would like to share with you a few points that made my family life easier during my doctorate. Although I have reflected specifically on my parental responsibilities here, there are a lot of translatable points. If you are perhaps caring for a parent, relative or friend alongside your doctoral commitments or you are a single parent, there are some nuggets here that you may find helpful.

General Tips

- *Be with them.* When you are with your children, be absolutely and completely with them. This means getting rid of your devices and computers and not thinking about your doctorate during this time. This will afford you the opportunity to invest in what is most important and will create some space between you and your studies. It will also make you feel that you are doing a good job!
- *Schedule it.* Define family time in advance so that both you and your children have something exciting to look forward to. I used a white board on the fridge to indicate to the children the days when we had some time together, the days when I was away and the days when I was home. In this way they had a visual cue as to when exciting things happened and when mummy needed to work. To this day I find this white board useful.
- *Keep it simple.* Time with your children does not need to be complicated. Often the best one-to-one time can involve something that needs to be done anyway, such as preparing a meal and eating and enjoying it together. Bedtime or story time also really helps to unwind at the end of the day. Let's face it, you can't think about anything else when you are bathing a child or reading a story, so it really helps to give your brain a break.
- *Be consistent.* Routine will really help you and your children. Routine rituals could include a Friday trip to the library or having pancake breakfast on Saturday. My children and I really enjoyed the rituals where everything slowed down, there was no rush and we could just take our time together. However, remember that if you promise anything, they will hold you to it, so try to be consistent where possible and carve time out for all routine events.
- *Schedule critical events well in advance.* I found it extremely useful to plan family holidays, appointments for vaccines or any critical family events well in advance. Doing this will help you to feel in control of your calendar and help you to resist overcommitting to your work. It will also give you time to plan your annual leave with your supervisor and research team.
- *Share your work with your children.* Sometimes my boys were curious about what happened when I entered my office. I often shared pictures of my laboratory or papers that I was working on with them. Don't underestimate the role model you are becoming. Share the journey with them. You will be surprised how your work ethic translates and just how infectious your curiosity is.
- *Create one-on-one time.* If you have more than one child, try to schedule alone time with each of them. People will often say that going for a walk with your child or going a trip together in the car helps children to verbalise concerns more easily. For a working parent or caregiver, getting to the core of any problems sooner rather than later is a good thing. However, the activity you select will depend on the age of your children. For younger children it might include a relaxed day together at home; for older children it could be a trip to a local café or museum or spending time with them on their homework.

- *Be OK with not getting it right.* Sometimes you just won't get it right, and this is OK. Sometimes there is no answer to a particular issue, no matter how much you reflect and try to do it better next time. Whatever the circumstance, remember that you are doing your best, and that as doctoral parents we all share similar journies.
- *Community is important.* For a parent or caregiver, community is extremely important, as it is very easy to feel isolated during the doctoral journey. Joining a group of fellow parents or creating your own group of like-minded academics who are going through a similar experience is useful. Throughout my doctorate, I met some amazing academic parents and caregivers whom I felt able to talk to. By reaching out to others, you will find that they experience the same challenges. Don't underestimate the power of connection; it can help to raise your spirits on very difficult doctoral days.
- *Use your annual leave.* To stay healthy and happy as a doctoral parent or care, it is important to avail yourself of all of your annual leave. Rest is important, and a break can really help to revitalise and motivate. If you have a few days to spare, pencil in a day of annual leave now and again to just be a parent. This helps when you need some time to take stock of what is happening in your own home. This could include cleaning your office space and files, organising the kids' clothes and school uniforms, thinking ahead of what might be required or getting a Christmas costume organised. In my experience, taking control in these simple ways can help to reduce anxiety and unclutter your mind, leaving you better able to focus on your doctoral work.
- *Create flexibility.* Think about flexible hours to meet your requirements. Are there opportunities to work from home or to work in a different way (five days in four days, for example)? Flexible working is usually negotiable with your employer and can really help you to feel on top of your family life. Don't be afraid to ask for what you need or to discuss the options with your doctoral supervisor.
- *Set expectations.* Undertaking a doctorate is all-encompassing but may be difficult for family or friends members to understand if we do not explain the commitments required. Take time with your partner, family or close friends to discuss the pressures, and regularly negotiate childcare plans that suit you and your family. Once the expectations are clear, in terms of the support you require or the demands on your time, you will avoid confusing and disappointing those close to you.
- *Avail yourself of any additional help.* If it is possible to get your shopping delivered or to share shopping or cleaning responsibilities, this can be a game changer. When you have young children, cleaning is a 24-hour job. I often struggled to 'do it all' and cleaned most of the weekends, which meant less time with my family. To avoid this, my husband and I agreed to share the housework and shopping in the first instance, but in the latter stages of my doctorate, I found online shopping and help from a local house cleaner extremely useful.

Childcare

For any working parent or caregiver, having childcare that works is very important. If you do not have childcare that you are happy with, it can really affect your focus and progress with your studies. Based on my experience so far, I suggest that taking time to consider and research the options is the best way forward. Although I cannot say that my experiences were entirely straightforward, reflecting the journeys of most parents, I hope that sharing some of my reflections will help to unmask some of the potential issues.

Many of my colleagues found that asking a family member or friend to assist with childcare was the best way forward. The benefits of your child knowing the caregiver and being in a familiar environment may help both you and your child as you take the initial step to return to work.

Also, the financial burden is usually less prohibitive. However, as with every childcare option, it is important to think through some of the potential cons:

- It may be more of a challenge to discuss things you are unhappy with due to the closeness of your relationship with a friend or family member.
- It may be more difficult to extend your hours or work out of office hours if you need to.
- If they are minding your child in their home, it will be more difficult to dictate the terms, such as who enters the house or not while your child is there. Indeed, this can be a problem with childcare that takes place in any childminder's home, so this is certainly something to consider, as this option will not be as regulated as a traditional nursery, where security, accountability and visiting are more tightly controlled.

More recently, some of my colleagues used shared parental leave, where it is possible to take a shared approach to childcare for the first 12 months. Although this was not an option for me at the time, many universities are becoming more flexible to support families so that childcare becomes less of a financial and practical burden. Therefore, prior to maternity leave, why not check out the options with human resources to see how the university can support you with this?

Hiring a childminder may also prove a viable option for those who do not have direct family support or the option for shared parental leave. When my children were extremely young, it was hard to imagine sending them off to nursery. I liked the thought of the children being able to stay in their home environment with their home comforts. Therefore, in the first instance, we decided to hire a local childminder who would work from our home.

Our childminder worked for a local nursery and had all the relevant paperwork and security checks complete. I interviewed our childminder together with my husband, reviewed her qualifications and references, and invited her for a trial day to see how she interacted with my children. It all seemed ideal and for the most part it was, until it was not. What I mean by this is that as much as you undertake background and qualification checks and interview your childminder, at the end of the day, childminders can let you down. They will be sick, they can let you down at the last moment, and in the end, this unpredictability affected my focus and my ability to do my work. This is also challenging because as the manager of a childminder, if things are not working out, you will need to address it, and this is not always easy. In a strange way, the relationship you will have with a childminder is rather like a marriage. If the fit is not correct, it will have an impact on you and your family and you will have to deal with it.

This experience led me to seek nursery care for my children, that is, care provided by a regulated provider. The regulated provider takes care of employing childminders who are qualified and vetted to undertake the role. I personally found this to be the best option for my family, as there was never a problem with sick leave or inconsistencies of any kind. This ultimately led to a more peaceful and calmer family life. The experience also benefitted my children, as they learned a lot from playing with other children. Provision of daily reports of what they had eaten and how they were feeling during the day also helped me to feel more in control and better able to concentrate on my work during the day.

One of the cons of nursery care may be the location. At the beginning, I did not quite understand how stressful it can be getting to a nursery on time for dropoffs or pickups. Nurseries usually have a strict timetable outside of which you will not be able to drop off your child or pick them up. This is important to consider and discuss directly with the nursery in advance. Unlike a live-in childminder, who may be more flexible and adaptable to different schedules, including situations where you are running late or need to leave early for work, it is my experience that nurseries are not. Therefore, in considering nurseries, it will be necessary to think about travel times and whether the location is realistic. I also found it useful to think about how I might travel to the nursery in the morning. For example, if I selected a nursery near my home, it meant that I did not have to bring my children on public transport through the city of London. An additional benefit was that once I had dropped the children off, my mental transition to work could begin and I could arrive ready for the day ahead.

However, some of my colleagues found it easier to bring their children directly to a university-based nursery. In this way, if their babies needed to be breast-fed or their children became ill, they were near enough to deal with the task at hand. Whether you choose a nursery close to your home or your university, I feel quite sure that it does not make a difference which you select as long as you consider all of the pros and cons relating to each option and discuss it as a family together so you feel settled as you return to your studies.

Despite these considerations, a rather unexpected benefit of nursery was that it really supported my children in transitioning to primary school. Since the children were familiar with waving me or my husband goodbye at the nursery door and were secure in the knowledge that we would return to collect them in the evening, it really helped. It supported the transition so well that on their first day at primary school, my children waved us off and cheerfully skipped in the door, leaving us sobbing at the school gate!

As children get older and gain independence, different options will become available to you, such as after-school clubs and activities. My elder now walks home from school and is capable of doing his homework independently, requiring guidance now and again. You will find that as your children get older, you will need to adapt your approach again and again. With experience, you will become confident in adopting and refining the approach to suit your child and family in the best way. At this point the financial burden of childcare becomes less and you will begin to see the fruits of your labour. You will realise that your work ethic and facilitation of independence were worth it and that your children are prepared well for future life experiences.

Although I have focused on childcare within this section, I have learned from my experiences of caring for my mother that being a caregiver for an ill relative also has the potential to place a huge burden on doctoral students. I have since heard people describing my generation as the sandwich generation; that generation where, just as your career takes off, your children remain dependent and your parents become ill. This is not easy. Again, it is important to acknowledge the support you need during this time, whether from relatives and friends or whether the situation requires you to avail yourself of home help or professional support.

Whatever your circumstances, with the right support, I would like to reassure you that your doctoral journey will be possible. With the right people to talk to, you will be able to navigate just about any hurdle you encounter. It is always a great comfort to share difficulties with those you trust, including family, friends or doctoral peers. Remember also that your supervisory team are there to support you, so do not be afraid to share any concerns with them as they are well placed to direct you towards specific support services that are available within the university, including pastoral care, financial services and human resources. They can also ensure confidentiality and discuss flexible options, such as a temporary leave of absence, to support you during these difficult times.

Dealing With Judgement

Dealing with judgement is perhaps one of the most difficult things for a parent or caregiver. It is something that I encountered more than once, but as I have grown in confidence as a parent and my children are older now, I find it to be less of a problem. It seems to me that the judgement of working parents comes thick and fast when children are younger, particularly from parents who have elected a different way of living and bringing up their children. I am not writing this to judge others but rather believe that we should all be able to stand strongly in what works best for us and our circumstances.

Comments from other parents could really hurt me at times. During my doctorate, I would make a deliberate point of attending the important events, including my children's concerts and parent–teacher evenings. I would deliberately carve time out in the diary to do so. However, in the interest of defending my time, I would also politely decline any invitations for events that were not so critical, such as parent coffee mornings, drinks or dinners. As a result, parents and teachers would see me now and again but not at all events and I was OK with this. However, one morning it appeared that they were not OK with my choices and decisions, as one parent spoke out loudly, 'Oh, so Samuel does have a mummy, then!' As she laughed, I found myself close to tears. It was so hurtful to me that they could think I was less of a parent because I chose not to drink with them until the early hours or go to parent social events. At that time my children were so small that such comments really affected my confidence in my choices. Perhaps the fact that I was not parenting as I had been parented and that I was carving a new way also affected my confidence. Why could I not stand strong in my choice?

It is possible that you will experience such judgements on your doctoral journey. However, I encourage you to stand strong in your decisions as you are finding your way. Remember the role model you are becoming for your children, remember your 'why'. There is no right way to be a parent, and no one will ever understand the expectations on your shoulders or the responsibilities you carry as a doctoral student. This is why their feelings about you or your actions are none of your concern. Surround yourself with like-minded individuals, of whom there will be many. Refresh and reaffirm yourself in the knowledge that you are doing what is right for you and your family and you will do this in your way.

Challenging Times

People's lives are never straightforward, and I am no exception to this. After the first year of my doctorate, I was blessed to have my second son. At this point, when I had two very young children, my mother was diagnosed with Parkinson's disease and my father with colon cancer. Throughout my doctorate, as my mother's symptoms advanced, I was also dealing with the heaviness that grief brings. The grief of gradually losing someone cannot be underestimated. It invaded my focus and wove its way through my days. At first I ignored my instinct to seek help, thinking that I could just deal with it. I thought that if I just worked harder, I could make it work—I could achieve amidst the heaviness of grief. However, the reality was that it was becoming a struggle to concentrate and focus. It was time to reach out for help.

The first person I approached was my main supervisor, and I also discussed it with colleagues. By discussing it openly with people I trusted, I was able to interrogate the issue and problem-solve. In the end, I received grief counselling, which really helped. It helped me to gain clarity that although my mum was still alive, I was in fact grieving for all that I was losing on a very gradual basis. Through the support of a grief counsellor, I realised that I could reframe my grief and use it as a driver for my work. I also imagined the grief that my patients experienced, their loss of ability and quality of life. I used my advocacy to drive change for the positive. My grief could be found in the words I wrote so passionately about patients, in the messages I disseminated at conferences, through creation of community and the determination I felt to change things for the better. In fact, it is in the very words that I am typing now. You cannot forget it, you cannot control it, so let it be your driver for good.

At one of the most challenging points of my doctoral journey, I recall being invited to talk at a European conference in Berlin. I had been working very hard that month and I was exhausted from overworking. To be honest, I was possibly entering burnout but did not realise it. As I entered the plane and sat in a solitary chair being asked if I would like tea or coffee by the air hostess, the guilt of leaving my two baby boys for the first time filled me. I began to question why I was doing this. Was this what a 'good parent' looked like? Was it worth it?

On arrival at the conference, I appeared to be the only delegate who was pre-doctoral, a female and not wearing a navy or black suit. They did not look like me and I was finding it difficult to see how I fitted into this world. It was quite an overwhelming experience, particularly for a new investigator. However, all I could think to do was to make sure that my conference poster was up and professionally presented and then wander around the vast European underground of what seemed like endless tunnels of scientific posters and researchers.

Then came the first presentation that I was interested in listening to. I decided to take a deep breath and claim the seat that I was invited there to take. Suddenly, the empathic tones of an extremely experienced clinical researcher filled the air around me. I believed she knew and understood what it felt like to be lost in a sea of academics. How grateful I was that she reached out and that she took the time to share her story of navigating being a mother on one hand and an academic on the other. I was no longer alone. Now as I support others in research, I recognise how powerful such simple gestures are. Maybe you can be this support for another? You may have doubts or fears, but don't underestimate the power of the shared experience.

By sharing experiences in this way, I felt encouraged to re-evaluate the way in which I organised my time. The old Janet would have made time for writing over the weekend, applied for grants in her lunch hour and forgotten about her personal pursuits in order to produce the best work. However, from this point on, I accepted that I could not work any harder. The old ways of working were no longer serving me as a parent, and I needed to make changes.

Take Care of Yourself

There was support out there, but I needed to search for it. My university had alerted me to two courses to support parents and caregivers in scientific research careers. Although I have since learned that there is no education that will completely furnish you with the plethora of skills you will require as a parent or caregiver, there was a lot of wisdom to be gained through these experiences. On reflection, perhaps the most important advice that I gained from these experiences was 'take care of yourself'. This mantra became useful during the difficult doctoral days, where you feel as if you are sinking with the personal and professional responsibilities that doctoral research inevitably brings.

At first, 'take care of yourself' seemed impossible, as taking care of myself was not my natural default position, whereas taking care of others was. I expect it is that we care for others that makes us ideally placed for careers as healthcare professionals. However, as I have observed, our typical default position of overworking at the expense of our health is an attribute shared by many academics. Early in my career, I learned that there was a unseen badge of honour to be gained from working through the night and weekends and not taking lunch. In fact, before I became a clinician, I even recall seeing a bed in one of the labs I worked in so that researchers could watch their bacteria through the night!

However, these ways of working will not serve you well during a doctorate. It is definitely a case of needing to put on your own life jacket before you attend to those of others, including family and friends. When it came down to it, asking simple questions of myself such as 'What do I need today?' really helped. For a parent or caregiver, it is often the very basic needs that are forgotten. Am I hungry? Am I tired? Do I need to take a 10-minute break before the next meeting to gather my thoughts? Do I need a cup of tea? Although a cultural shift is required and the landscape is very gradually changing, I believe there is room for us to all lead by example so that we have what we need to advance as leaders in research alongside our personal commitments.

The question I have been asked the most by fellow parents and caregivers in healthcare research is how one creates an effective work/life balance. To this the answer is quite simply, I am still learning. As your children grow and caring needs change, there is a need for continual reappraisal. When I returned to my doctoral research 6 months after the birth of my second son, I did so because I feared that I would not be able to return or have the confidence required to return if I left it any longer. At this point, my children were so young that I found it difficult to leave the house in the morning. They were completely dependent upon me, but I really enjoyed my work and needed to return. During this stage, it was necessary to have support in place to pave the way for a successful return. As I did not know of anyone within the university who had been on a similar journey, it really helped when the university facilitated engagement with other parents in a similar position. Research is such a specific career with so many demands and pressures that I needed to be within a community that understood my journey and to which I could relate. I remember the first meeting vividly, so many exhausted parents having had only two or three hours of sleep, luxuriating in the time they now had to think about what was actually going on in their lives. It was a chance to debrief and let it all out. There I sat among physicists, healthcare professionals, neuroscientists and computer analysts, a veritable patchwork quilt of leading researchers who had lost their way and needed to find it.

Meeting With Myself

During this meeting, we all shared techniques that we found helpful. One that I shared, I like to call 'meeting with myself'. Although this sounds quite selfish, in reality it was the only way I found to survive the transition from my home life, in which I was mother, wife and caregiver, to my research life, in which I was undertaking a funded PhD fellowship with associated deadlines and expectations. This 'meeting with myself' helped me to transition from Mother mode to Researcher mode. As I travelled to work most days on the bus, there was little time to be on my own. I would usually use this time to connect dutifully with the news of the day, double-check that all was all right at home and quickly check my e-mails. Once the bus ride finished, I would then walk to my favourite coffee shop, about 12 minutes from my workplace. I would order my favourite cup of tea and take the time to sit in my own chair, uninterrupted by little hands and voices. During my 'meeting with myself' I would take out my well-thumbed moleskin journal and my favourite pen and would use the time to write. I would write all of the things that I needed to consider for the day, the priorities for my research, the priorities for my home life and the bits of me that I had forgotten. This ritual enabled me to create order from disorder as I transitioned from one life to another. As I shared this ritual with others at the meeting, I understood that many researchers related to this issue. It was not an experience that was peculiar to me or my profession; it affected everyone.

It's Good Enough

As the meeting continued, the facilitators shared their own personal stories of how they navigated busy jobs alongside the commitment of parenthood. Their journey was also extremely relatable. I slowly realised that the pursuit of perfection as a working parent or caregiver is a particularly fruitless exercise, as there are too many variables to control. Kids get sick, childcare breaks down, clothes need to be washed and houses to be cleaned. Aiming for perfection at any level is simply too restrictive and places you in a permanent position of failure. However, if we reframe this as 'it's good enough', suddenly everything becomes that little bit lighter and brighter. Suddenly, that paper that you have lovingly redrafted for the tenth time becomes acceptable and 'good enough' to submit after the first revision or the chapter of your doctoral thesis that you feel unable to part with, you can let go of and share with your supervisors. You realise that neither your research nor your home deserves to gleam more brightly than you and your family.

Partnership

However, there was another important lesson that I would like to share. In order for any research journey to succeed, everyone needs to be on board. Before undertaking my doctoral research, I worked as a teaching fellow at King's College London. This was a great experience to learn from academics in a related field, but in particular to learn from colleagues with parental and caring responsibilities. I recall a compulsion I had to ask everyone about their experiences of parenthood as an academic in order to lock this down and be a parent in the 'best' way possible. As I was the first woman in my family to undertake doctoral studies, there was no guiding light, so I needed to find my own. I recall reaching out to one of the academics that I related to most, and she kindly and candidly shared her journey. I remember her instructing me that it was of the utmost importance to let my partner experience it all; 'let your partner parent and care, let your partner succeed and fail'.

Although letting someone fail seemed harsh to me at the time, it seemed that in order to work well as a team, all contributors to childcare needed to be on the same page, so that each person had the capacity to contribute effectively. However, the only way in which a contributor can contribute well is if they have the skills. Therefore, letting go of the control of feeding or cooking, for example, and inviting others to contribute no matter what the outcome (failure or success) meant that contributors were happy to learn the skills they required without fear of judgement. In my experience, giving my partner the opportunity to fail increased his confidence as a parent, reduced his reliance on me as the sole childcare provider and improved our family dynamics. The result was that our children knew that they could rely equally on both of their caregivers, and we avoided complete burnout.

When I began my doctorate, my husband had just set up his own business. It was what he had always dreamed of doing, and in an effort to support each other's dreams, we agreed that there was no time like the present and that financially we would be able to support our family during this transition. However, I failed to realise just how much work this would require. Having a young family and just starting out in my PhD, I began to feel the squeeze. Late nights, nursery dropoffs, losing our connection because we were like ships in the night, were a few of the real challenges we were faced with.

There was also the extreme guilt I would feel if the kids were ill and I needed time off to look after them. At the beginning, I would take the time off, as my husband earned more than I and I feared that if his business failed it would affect the family. However, great counsel from my supervisors and friends made me understand that it is important to share such responsibilities. From this point on and to this day, we work in partnership to share parental responsibility so that we may all thrive.

No-Responsibility Nights

However, culturally, sharing parental responsibilities may not always be acceptable. From my personal experience of growing up in Ireland, these rules of equity between working parents did not always seem to apply. The job of the mother was to look after the kids and the job of the father to provide. As a child I quickly learned that mothers take on an inordinate number of tasks, but rather than these being shared, Mothers take over because it's 'just easier to do it myself'. However, I have learned that this strategy is not so useful for an academic. As a doctoral student, you need to be able to share the parental responsibilities. This approach has made a world of difference to me and my family. It also resulted in 'no-responsibility nights' where we gave each other one night with freedom from all parental responsibilities each week. In this way we could remember who we were as individuals, catch up with friends, exercise or simply rest. When the weight of total responsibility lifts, everything becomes that little bit lighter. It becomes easier to breathe, to rest and refresh completely.

Final-Year Frankness

The final year of a doctorate is busy. Although you will have worked hard from the beginning and may have everything in order, nerves undoubtedly begin to kick in. It feels like freewheeling down a mountain: There is no way back and you need to face forward and embrace it all as you approach the finish line. For a parent or caregiver, this may place relations with family, friends and partners under strain.

However, it is possible to minimise this strain through frank communication. In the final year this is critical, as you will have deadlines to meet and require pure focus. At the beginning of my final year, I recall sitting down with my husband in order to prepare him. I engaged with him on the frankest level that I have ever spoken with anyone. I shared that my final year was the culmination of years of work and that the outcome was extremely important to me and my future career. I charted out what the year could look like in terms of the time I would need to write and the requirement to work some weekends or early mornings. However, I also made it clear that I would commit to non-negotiable family time at the weekends and every evening. Because I did so, there were then no unpleasant surprises when it came to needing time to write at the weekends or to go to the library, since the stage was set and my needs were clear from the beginning. To this day our schedules are continually evolving and changing; however, with regular communication and the use of shared diaries, we rarely experience too many unexpected surprises that affect our work and family life.

Pay It Forward

Having successfully navigated the doctoral process as a parent, I like to share what I have learned with those who are beginning to travel the same path. I think that for academic parents and caregivers who have successfully achieved it is important to pay our learning forward. I believe it is the responsibility of all parents in academic fields to share our knowledge and to use our words of encouragement for the next generation. After all, it is in those words that people find the greatest comfort. You will never know how much an inspirational message, nudge or gesture means until you experience it as a doctoral student. Now as I travel on in academia, I have begun to understand how important it is to listen and be open to the universe, to take in all of the positive, to remember all of the elements that helped me on my way and to share these.

Ask for the Flexibility You Need

Since graduating, I have been approached many times to discuss how to prepare for a doctorate as a caregiver or parent. Although all of the elements I have discussed so far are important, perhaps the most intuitive but not so well-executed strategy for healthcare professionals in research is to feel comfortable with setting firm boundaries. When I started my doctorate I became pregnant, and recognising the work involved in having two kids under the age of three years old at home, while undertaking research at a top research university, filled me with dread. In my laboratory, nobody had ever taken maternity leave; in fact, I was one of the first healthcare professionals in research outside of medicine to undertake a research role within this particular laboratory. The anxiety of potentially not being able to deliver was more than I could bear.

However, I was extremely fortunate to have an amazing supervisor. She helped me to remember my 'why': why I was in this, why I deserved to continue. At this point I realised that supervisors understand that the road is not easy, they know you have been selected because of your determination, application, motivation and intellectual abilities, and they believe that you already have it in you to succeed. Therefore, from a supervisor's perspective, as long as you get your work done, for the most part, it does not matter where this happens or if the schedules need to change or the working hours need honing. This is all up for negotiation, and it is your job as a doctoral student to recognise this and to ask for the flexibility you require to make things work.

Boundaries and Goals

With the support of my supervisor and team, I returned to work following 6 months of maternity leave. Although I definitely needed a year with my first child, this was my second experience of motherhood, and so I felt able and ready to return earlier. Upon my return, I began by placing distinct boundaries between my work and home life. Initially this consisted of entering the workplace at 8 am to check e-mails, to plan and to get a head start on the day. I found that this really helped me to set the agenda for the day ahead and even to do some writing if I felt so inclined, as the office was quiet at this time. I would then use the rest of the day to, for example, attend meetings, undertake research, support students or write. In general, I found scheduling and setting goals for each day was really important. In academia, everything can take on a somewhat nebulous frame. This lack of structure may be difficult for healthcare professionals making the transition to academia, as it seems there is no agenda, no timeline and no schedule. However, what you soon realise is that at this level of study, your day is entirely self-directed. Feeling uncomfortable without goals, I applied what I knew to help productivity in practice. I decided to set specific goals during my 'meeting with myself' each morning. This way, it did not matter if the day went well or it did not; I could still achieve my baseline targets. As I like to write and put pen to paper, I liked to create a list in my favourite notebook each day. However, this list could be created in any format or way you wish, so do what works best for you. Once my targets were achieved, there was simply nothing better than checking each item off the list!

To create boundaries, I also invested in some noise reduction headphones for the office. I cannot tell you what a difference this made. Headphones not only help you to concentrate but also give a message to your colleagues that you are focusing on important work and that you are not to be disturbed. Delightfully, my team embraced me and my headphones. In addition, my headphones really helped at home when I needed to work in nontraditional workspaces while my kids were playing. In doctoral and post-doctoral research, there are certainly times as a parent when you need to focus, and the only way this can happen is by creating the possibility of peaceful moments. Somehow you need to find your way, and you do. You will find that you become creative and innovative in the approaches you take and that this adaptability will serve you well in the rest of your academic career.

Finding Your Way Now and in the Future

I am very fortunate to have had a great community of academic colleagues, who regularly shared their thoughts with me and offered advice. Although we all found the space, time and peace we needed to complete our doctorates, we did it in different ways. It is important to remember that there is no right way when it comes to being a doctoral parent or caregiver; your own way is enough. In the end it's all about creating opportunity where there seems to be none. You will be surprised by how creative you become when you do not have the luxury of time.

As your children grow or your caring responsibilities change, different approaches will be required. Simultaneously, your career will progress with new demands and expectations. While undertaking a doctorate, you may be driven by the apprenticeship of acquiring new knowledge, learning new methodologies and producing a thesis; in post-doctoral research you will begin to hone your skills, focus your research agenda and prepare for leadership. However, don't underestimate the life skills that you will acquire on the journey. Once it has been navigated, you will realise with the benefit of time that the doctoral journey is much more than an apprenticeship in research; it is an apprenticeship in life skills that you will use and share for the benefit of others in the future.

Finding Your Way The Doctoral Parent and Caregiver – Learning Points

- Don't worry about being the perfect parent or caregiver. It is OK to be 'good enough' in all aspects.
- Take time to be with those you care for. Get rid of devices and computers and invest in time together.
- Schedule time to connect. Give yourself and your family a date to look forward to. Create one on one time with your children where possible. This may help you to pick up any issues sooner rather than later.
- The simple things matter. You may not have time to go on day trips or outings but don't discount the simple things. Preparing a meal together or sharing story time can be equally enriching and may also give your brain some much needed rest.
- Schedule critical events such as holidays or doctor appointments in advance. This will avoid disappointment and keep you and your family safe and healthy.
- Share your work with those you care for. Never underestimate the inspiration you are or the role model you are becoming.
- Community is important. Don't feel isolated. Reach out to fellow academics, local group or create your own group to support you on your doctoral journey.
- Ask for what you need. Discuss options with human resources or your supervisor in terms of flexible working or childcare. To avoid disappointment and frustration, set expectations in advance with family, friends or childcare providers.
- Take the time to consider your childcare options in advance of returning to work and negotiate a return to work option that suits you best.
- When the old ways of working are no longer serving you, change them.
- Place boundaries between work life and home life and stick to them. Don't forget your noise reduction headphones!
- Share your story and pay your experiences forward. Don't underestimate the difference you can make.

Finding Your Way: The Doctoral Parent and Caregiver – Action Points

The most important action points that I can act on today/this week/this month are

Finding Your Way: The Doctoral Parent And Caregiver – Steps Towards Achieving Action Points

The next steps I can take towards these action points are

CHAPTER 9

Academic Writing

I kept writing. I kept not getting published, but it was okay,
because I was getting educated.
—Elizabeth Gilbert

One of the elements that I perhaps did not appreciate at the beginning of my doctorate was exactly how much time I would spend writing: writing abstracts for conferences, writing for publication, writing presentations and applications for small grants to fund collaborative work. Writing does not always come easy. It is a skill that takes practice. Writing requires patience, space and time, all of which are in short supply for a parent, caregiver or clinical researcher.

As a clinician, it is common to feel that perhaps your writing is not good enough. Maybe you have lost your confidence with academic writing, as you have not been needed to write in an academic way for a while, or perhaps you never had any confidence in academic writing in the first place. Although I had completed an MSc in advance of my doctorate, I mistakenly believed that I would need to complete a course in academic English literature before I could ever become an educated writer. However, I am here to reassure you that although there may be merit in education to some degree, in my experience, the education lies very much in the doing. In other words, if you wish to get better at academic writing, you just need to write!

Writing Habits

It is important to recognise that writing, especially with regard to larger pieces of work such as a doctoral thesis, takes time. In the beginning it is a matter of simply taking baby steps in the direction of your final goal. As James Clear points out in his book *Atomic Habits* (see Resources), it is important to cast a vote in the direction in which you wish to travel. So if your end goal is to publish a journal article or to begin writing your thesis, cast votes in that direction through consistent writing practice.

Casting votes in the right direction will look differently for different people. As I engaged with different academics and clinical researchers, I realised that in the early stages before my research had started, writing could simply include reflective pieces in journals or professional magazines, abstracts for conferences, case reports or writing up planned research protocols and submitting them for publication. Small beginnings such as protocols can be used as platforms on which to lay out the beginnings of your thesis chapters. Indeed, small beginnings can feel like mini wins, serving to motivate you. Often, it's the simple things that move you forward. Anything from writing bullet points on a page from which to plan an abstract or laying out subheadings for a potential article can be incredibly motivating. Somehow there is something special and amazingly satisfying about no longer dealing with blank pages!

When you write, it is important that you have freedom in it. By this I mean that you are not writing for anyone other than yourself, that you submerge yourself in your 'why' and give yourself permission to lock out the outside world. This freedom means that you avoid second guessing yourself or thinking of what everyone else may think about your words and your reflections. This freedom means that you can enter a writing state, in which the words will almost come faster that you can type them, and it becomes easier to write thesis chapters or a paper. Some authors refer to this as the 'flow state' or as screenplay writer Shonda Rhimes refers to it, the 'hum'.

When you are in the 'hum', you do not need to limit yourself with punctuation or by continuously spell checking or rephrasing everything. In this way you can be free, and the words will simply come. Before you know it, that blank page becomes filled with words and outlines, giving you confidence that you can do this. The act of writing itself drives you forwards, and the education very much comes with the writing. As Elizabeth Gilbert alludes to in her writing (see the Resources section), to become a better writer you need to go ahead and write.

Habitual writing became important to me at the start. It is interesting how the brain works. Initially I began writing whenever I found the opportunity. As a mum of young children, I remember, I would grab any small bits of time I had to just write. However, I soon recognised that writing at different times of day was challenging, mainly because my brain just wasn't always 'writing ready'. Therefore, I needed to develop a writing habit. As I am a morning person, I found setting aside a consistent time to write every day to be extremely helpful. To be completely honest and share openly with you, when my kids were young, I used to wake up at 4.30 a.m. so that I could have an hour of writing time while the house was quiet. My husband thought I was crazy, but honestly this time was like a golden hour: no noise, no interruptions, just pure writing freedom.

However, this golden hour may look different for each of you. Therefore, I very much hope that through sharing my approach you will begin to find the way that suits you and your lifestyle best. My ideal scenario was always to write at the same time and to write every day. I have later learned that there is something in that habit. By writing every day you are training your brain and your subconscious to be writing ready at the same time each day, almost like training your body when it needs breakfast or requires exercise. A consistent habit really helped.

Before I began, I liked to make sure that my desk was clear of potential distractions, removing my mobile phone, extraneous books and paperwork. I would fill a glass of water and make a hot cup of tea and place them within hand's reach. I used my favourite desk lamp in order not to alert the little ones that I was up and ready for action. It was my one chance to get on top of the day. It meant that no matter how the rest of the day went, at least the beginning would always start as well as possible. This is obviously the ideal scenario; however, it did not always look like this based on how I felt or logistics. It is important to remember that not every day will work out in the way you plan, but at least you are trying to cast your vote towards your goal.

As a naturally curious person, I have also learned greatly from research colleagues who shared their stories along the way. Each person experienced their own personal challenges, but none the less, they did not let them deter them from their deserved success. Some of my research friends would write in their cars after dropping their kids off at football or found nuggets of time on public transport or while waiting in a dentist's waiting room. If you have your computer or paper and pen with you, it really can be as you define it. I have always found it amazing how these snatched minutes of time really work in my favour in the end. You would be surprised how much you can achieve in five to ten minutes a day, if this is all you have some weeks.

In fact, writing in small bursts of time can really add up. Although it is not quite enough to get into the flow of things sometimes, remember that there is always something you can do. Yes, more time definitely permits more writing depth; however, shorter blocks can be useful. For example, could you start writing your table of contents or do a spell check on the writing you did the day before? Are your references up to date and synchronised? Could you begin to use bullet points to put together a chapter outline? Remember that all these small bursts add up, and on a day when writing is not coming easily, there will always be a graph that needs to be altered or a reference that needs to be found. This approach is important to remember on difficult days.

As my house was usually a busy place and my work environment was open plan, I found the university library to be a quiet space in which to write. This was mainly because in the library I could be surrounded by like-minded individuals undertaking similar doctoral work. It gave me the feeling that we were all in it together, which at times was a great comfort and made me feel less isolated. Undertaking a doctorate can be an extremely isolating and lonely experience at times, so when you feel this way, it is important to recognise it and to change your environment.

If you have a shared office, it is often not easy to find a quiet space to write. I worked from an open plan office and found this a challenge. It was a great space in which to share ideas and discuss research, but not so great when it came to writing. In the beginning, I recall feeling increasingly on edge when writing in this environment. As what I like to call a highly functioning introvert, I find I get my energy from peaceful and quiet spaces. So quite quickly, I appreciated that I needed to change my environment when writing without completely isolating myself. Don't get me wrong, I enjoyed having my colleagues around me, to share a cup of tea or to catch up on their latest work; however, when it came to writing, I needed complete peace. To this end, it seemed to me that there was simply nothing else for it than a pair of the biggest, pilotlike noise reduction headphones that the world or my lab had ever seen. They were large and ugly, but at this point I did not care. It was what I needed to be productive, and so I wore them with pride. Looking back, I am quite sure that everyone must have thought I looked hilarious. However, it did not bother me; I needed them. Later I would learn that there were also some secondary benefits. First, when I put the headphones on, it meant that people understood that I was writing and knew that I did not wish to be disturbed; but second, the act of putting them on was almost like a Pavlovian dog experiment in which the silence signalled to my brain, 'It's time to write,' and so I did. Honestly, they were the best investment. I must confess that I even used them in our apartment when I needed to write and my two little boys wanted to watch children's television. In this way I could observe them but did not need to hear Peppa Pig jumping up and down in muddy puddles as I sorted out my reference lists or did other such simple tasks. In the end, my headphones became part of my anatomy. We were inseparable!

Writing Support

As you begin to write, you may feel an urge to attend a writing course, but don't forget that you are educating yourself in every word you write and every phrase you thoughtfully arrange. During my doctorate I learned that writing is writing. No matter what your profession or background, the challenges and the failures are similar. Therefore, reading outside of my scope of practice helped to get a not so stuffy perspective on writing and authorship. As I have learned from such authors as Elizabeth Gilbert, whose book I reached for when I became more curious about writing (see the Resources section), it is not always necessary to attend a course to learn how to write, but writing practice is essential and support useful.

Writing support comes in many ways, and during my doctorate I learned that if the support was not there, then I would simply create it. Most universities have free writing courses available to you as part of your academic registration. Some of these may be superficial; others have depth to them, so it is important to gauge what level of support you require, where you are in the doctoral process, and to gain feedback from previous attendees or fellow doctoral students as to which course may be best for you so that you are not wasting time and are maximising your progress.

One of the courses that I found most beneficial was a university-led writing retreat. To attend the retreat, the university required that you were in the final year of your doctorate. They set the expectations very clearly from the beginning so that you understood that this was a quiet writing retreat, where you would make writing progress and have access to academic writing support as required. It was extremely helpful. It involved one overnight stay in a stately home in the middle of the English countryside. For that one weekend, I was able to shed all of the distracting forces and truly focus on my writing. The solitude and space made a great difference to my writing, but more interestingly, I found that being in a community of doctoral students really motivated me. Moving forward, I knew I needed to create a similar space for myself, and so I did, in my way.

In the United Kingdom at the time, it appeared that there were not many health care professionals undertaking further education at the doctoral level. At the time I began in the laboratory, where I started my PhD, I was the only clinician. Therefore, I decided to reach out to try and connect with others in a similar position. I began to create a research community. At first, we met in person, and during this time, I decided to begin mini-writing retreats. I asked one of my very kind mentors whether we could use a clinical meeting room within the hospital where we could write. When the department agreed for us to use this space, it unlocked a writing retreat possibility whenever we needed it, and so now and again, when motivation was waning for us all, we would get together and write.

One cannot underestimate the power of writing with others. When there is pure focus and you can trust the group to be as focussed as you are, there is simply nothing better. We would start each session by saying what we wanted to achieve, we would work for an hour or so, and then at the end we would reflect on what we had achieved and the challenges we had. In my experience, community can help you navigate most things, so if you feel that you don't have support, why not create your own community?

Of course, all of this is possible virtually also. During my doctorate, I met with other clinical researchers using trusted platforms. One person would agree to lead the session, at the beginning of which, we would share our ambitions for the time we had together. After turning off our cameras and pressing Mute, we would then write for an hour or so. Once the hour was up, with the cameras and sound on, we then fed back to each other regarding our progress. This is a nice thing to do when you have a trusted bunch of colleagues with whom you can share the ups and downs of your doctoral journey. Networking early on in your doctoral journey can really spark these opportunities, and sometimes you will find yourself creating and leading new things to take one step closer to achieving your intended goal. This has since led to the creation of a virtual community for health care professionals in research. So really, the sky is the limit. Remember, if community is not out there for you, create it.

Learning Needs

During the doctorate, you will learn so much about yourself you did not realise before. For example, I learned that I get my energy from being on my own and that after a lengthy conference I really need to spend some time in my own company to refresh myself. I also learned that with regard to writing I enjoyed routine and needed space and time to reflect. In the end, these insights really helped me: They enabled me to perform at my best and to communicate my needs to others. In the same way, it is possible that you may find that your learning needs relate to writing. This may not be obvious to you at the beginning but may be emphasized through the feedback you receive or through gradual inklings you get with time. You might find it difficult to read the text to inform your writing or to compose academic prose, perhaps because English is not your first language. Once you are aware of what the problem is and you feel able to share it in confidence with your supervisor, a trusted colleague or the university disability support services, you are on the way to sorting out the problem. Disability support services may put a plan of action in place, including reasonable adjustments to support you and your learning in the best way. Be brave and share your difficulties; you will be surprised at how much weight will be lifted off your shoulders through the support and resources you are offered. We are all different and academia is slowly changing to embrace this through the support it offers students. This is because academia recognises that it is through people's differences that the good stuff comes; your difference will set you apart from the rest.

Difficult Writing Days

Writing does not always come easy. In fact, people in the business of writing often refer to 'writer's block' as a period during which one just cannot write, through either lack of motivation or personal circumstance. When I began writing my thesis, I waited and wondered when my block would kick in and thought unhelpfully of the consequences that this may have for my doctoral writing. However, as I progressed, I began to learn that 'block' is not really an appropriate term. In fact, I would prefer to refer to it as 'writer's wake-up'. What I mean by this is that you need to let a difficult writing day, where you feel as if you cannot write or you do not have the motivation to write, become your 'wake-up'. When you get to the point where you are aware that today or this hour is going to be a challenging time to write, simply think about what your body is trying to tell you. This wake-up is your body's way of letting you know that something needs to change to continue.

When writing my thesis, I encountered many days where I found it difficult to write and I definitely needed to wake up or become alert to what my body needed. This will look differently for everyone and is why it is important to become aware of the circumstances that surround your 'wake-up'. To prompt this, I found it useful to ask myself one simple question 'what do I need right now?'. By asking yourself this question you should be open to meeting this need head on. It is important to be extremely honest with yourself in this situation and give yourself what you need.

In my case, my wake-ups often related to overworking. I would wake up early most mornings to write, put in a full day of work, spend time with the kids, take care of the house at night, and then continue to work again in the evening. On a repeated basis, this becomes tiring, and quite rightly, your body will tell you so. However, it is sometimes difficult to yield to these signs, as sometimes it feels as if when you are inspired to write you need to just go with it, especially when you are in the flow of it all.

When I was in a flow state, I embraced it and wrote until I literally could not write any more. I recall that my bedside notebook was sometimes filled with notes as ideas began to flow during the night. This sometimes happens when you are in the writing phases. Ideas come, and unless you commit them to paper, it can be extremely difficult to get a night's sleep. However, that said, don't discount the power of recording your writing ideas in your own way. A notebook can also be an extremely useful way of offering inspiration when you are less than motivated.

At some points, ideas and writing thoughts will come to you when you least expect them, so it's important to go with your flow and record them in some way that suits you—for example, writing them down or saving them as voice notes. Indeed, if you think best while walking, simply record your ramblings as you walk. There is some great voice recording software out there. In some ways, this may be less exhausting as you are simply free to record your ideas without feeling the need to punctuate every sentence or wonder how it might look on the page. In this way, you can embrace your flow while enjoying the benefits of exercise in the open air.

Although writing tends to flow best when one is relaxed and writing practice is consistent, there are occasions when you hit the wall. I found this to be the case when I entered the heavier writing phases. During these phases, you can almost feel the panic when the usual routine is no longer working for you, and therefore it is extremely important to be kind to yourself and wake up to your personal needs when this is the case.

Although there is no right way to attend to your needs, I would like to share with you some of the ways I learned to focus on difficult writing days. I really believe it is important to plan these, if possible, so that you gain the maximum benefit; you can look forward to the activity, use these moments to reward yourself for all that you do and enjoy the outcome. Here are some tips to support you:

- Take a break when you need it. This will be dependent on how much time you have, but mini-breaks often help. One of my friends used to take a cold shower when working from home to invigorate.

- Change environment. Is it possible to work from the library, home, a café or a friend's house?
- Remove distractions. Clean your desk by removing all potential distractions, turn all phone and computer notifications off and use a focussed screen option if this is available to you.
- Reward yourself once you reach your writing target for the day. Plan an activity that you enjoy: Meet up with friends, go food shopping or go for a walk in the fresh air while listening to your favourite podcast.
- Listen to relaxing music as you write. Often music without any words is the most helpful, but there are also a myriad of free music compilations available that use alpha waves and the like to increase focus. In fact, when I wanted to feel as if I were in a library and I could not get there, I listened to background library noises, which I enjoyed.
- Work with people if you feel isolated. There is something about the shared journey that can be motivating. Meet with a friend and work together.
- Arrange your own writing retreat. A colleague of mine booked a holiday to the Bahamas to finish her thesis and to find focus away from the teaching environment in which she worked. Although this is an extreme example, and was not something I could consider, it helps to get away. In my case, my holiday included visiting my parents' house or visiting my favourite library consistently.
- Identify the time of day when you write at your best and try to write at this time. For example, if you are an early bird like me, then habitually writing in the morning should work best for you. A writing routine really helps to create a flow state.
- Applications can be helpful. Certain apps, for example, use time as a motivational writing tool. Simply set the timer for the time you have available to write, and once the time is up, the app will set off an alert. If you do not have access to a similar app, simply set a timer.
- Take care of your health and well-being (see Chapter 7, Health and Well-Being).

Remember that you may also find it difficult to write on days when you have lots of meetings, phone calls or practical activities planned, such as laboratory or organisational work. This was my experience. If this is the case for you, too, simply recognise these days in advance and try to fit all related activities in on the same day. In this way, you will have days that are more writing-focussed and days that are more meeting- or talking-focussed. This will improve your efficiency. Although inevitably life will get in the way of the best laid plans, I recommend acknowledging the way in which you work best and taking control.

Step Away from the Writing

Sometimes no matter what you try, it just is not happening. If this is the case, I use the phrase 'step away from the writing' quite often. Acknowledging that you are not in flow as soon as possible is important. Otherwise, you are quite simply wasting your time. On these days you could bang your head on a brick wall and nothing would change. However, if you identify it early, you can simply recognise the day for what it is—not a writing day. Then you can move on and choose to be productive in another way or simply take a break.

Remembering Your 'Why'

As I mentioned earlier in the chapter, when I began to write, I often read the books of writers outside my scope of practice, as I simply did not wish to read another book that felt like reading an academic journal. During your doctorate it often feels this way. Since your doctoral work requires reading so many journals, when you take a break and read outside of your doctoral work, it may be difficult to read anything other than a newspaper or a magazine. I sought to read authors who wrote in non-academic language to understand the real story, the real nuts and bolts of writing.

Indeed, this has influenced the way I am writing this book, the book I needed to read when I was a doctoral student.

One such writer was the renowned author Elizabeth Gilbert. You may remember her writing from books such as *Eat, Pray, Love*, but one of her most recent writings struck a chord with me, and I have subsequently found a related podcast that she dedicates to the discussion of writing and solving writing problems (see the Resources section). When you read this book or listen to the podcast, you realise that you are not alone in the writing stakes and that every author, which is what you are now becoming, has writing issues that need to be resolved.

One of the quotations from her book entirely resonated with me. When I was young, my father always encouraged me to work hard. Indeed, he set the example. However, from Gilbert's work and my own experience of writing, you soon realise that hard work does not guarantee anything. This is difficult, because you assume that if you work really hard, you can navigate anything. However, on difficult writing days, it really does not matter how hard you work; the reward never seems to match the effort required to put words on the page. Sometimes we need to reframe our efforts, and by this I mean remembering your 'why'. This can be a powerful tool. If you cannot write for yourself, maybe you can write for the patients you serve. Maybe this 'why' is the most important driver; after all, it is why you are a clinician and it is why you are striving to do your research. Perhaps, if we begin to frame things in the love of what we do and why we are doing it, it will make it that bit easier and a lighter weight to carry. As Gilbert reassures us, sometimes 'hard work guarantees you nothing' but 'when it's for love, you will do it anyhow'.

Finding Your Way: Writing — Learning Points

- Remember that the more you write, the more educated and skilled you are becoming.
- Each university will offer a range of writing support, so check out what's available and what suits you best and ask previous attendees what their experience was or for their recommendations.
- Start writing early in your doctorate. Is there a protocol paper you could write, an abstract that you could plan to submit or a paper that you could contribute to or begin to write?
- Develop your writing ritual. Consider the time of day and environment in which you will work best.
- Accept that sometimes the stars will not align and that you may need to steal moments where you can, in a coffee shop, in the car or during a break in clinic. This is all OK because you are being consistent: you are committed to writing and doing it in the way that works best for you. You will be amazed how much small nuggets of time add up.
- If you have learning needs in relation to writing, it is important to identify them early on. You will be surprised how supportive universities are in this regard. Ask your supervisor or disability support services at your university who will be able to point you in the right direction.
- Writing does not have to be a lonely activity. Simply by changing your environment, creating a writing community or joining a writing group, you may feel less isolated and more motivated to write.
- If you cannot write, wake up to what might be happening. Be aware of what your needs are and attend to them.
- Step away from the writing. If you are not able to write on a particular day, step away from it and do something different. There is always something that you can do to move you forward in your research, and it is not always writing.
- Remember your 'why' to motivate you. Why are you doing this doctorate? What difference will your research make to your patients? What impact will it have?

Finding Your Way: Writing — Action Points

The most important action points that I can act on today/this week/this month are

Finding Your Way: Writing — Steps Towards Achieving Action Points

The next steps I can take towards these action points are

CHAPTER 10

Thesis Writing

Learning how to learn is life's most important skill.
—Tony Buzan

A doctoral thesis is essentially a book that you are required to write as part of the final examination. This book reflects all of the research you have undertaken as part of your doctorate and essentially sets the scene for your final oral examination or viva. At university there is usually a lot of writing support available for doctoral students. During my doctoral experiences some of the courses provided included the ones entitled 'Shut up and write' and 'Just write!' I recall thinking that the titles seemed quite harsh and directive. To be absolutely honest, they sounded like writing clubs that I did not want to be part of, like the writing equivalent of military-style fitness classes where they shout at you and say, 'Lie down on the floor and give me ten!'

However, upon reflection, and knowing what I know now, I realise how important this approach is when writing a thesis. If you wish to write a thesis, you are never 'ready'. If you wish to write a thesis, you need to just write.

Read a Thesis

In my experience, it is extremely important to practice writing from the very beginning of your doctorate and to take every opportunity to hone your skills. At the beginning of my doctorate many people, including academics and clinicians, advised me to read a bound thesis. At the time, I had never seen one. I presumed a thesis would look like something housed in my very favourite place, the British library, where the smell of aged paper and old leather surrounds the sacred texts housed within this church of books. I often felt intimidated by the size of some of these leather-bound books as they stood proudly within glazed casing, signalling a depth of knowledge that almost seemed out of reach. Therefore, it seemed quite a scary prospect to open and read a beautifully bound thesis with the thought of knowing that one day I would need to produce one. However, in hindsight, it was the best thing that I could have done.

I was very fortunate that my university had a shared portal of open-access theses from previous graduates. My lead supervisor also had some bound copies on her shelf that she was happy to share with me. I recall tentatively opening these theses to discover everything I needed to know. It helped me to understand the layout, the order of a thesis, the standard of writing required and how a thesis could be a personalised and unique contribution. It was inspiring and unbelievable to think that this is where I was headed. However, by now I understood that the train had already left the station. I realised that the time had come. I was about to write my first book.

In the early stages it felt as if writing a thesis was an insurmountable challenge, especially when you begin to appreciate the required word count, which varies between universities but can be up to 100,000 words or more in some cases. Although, at first reading, a thesis may make you feel like running in the opposite direction, take courage, engage and be inspired by these books of doctoral success. When reading a thesis, it does not matter that you do not understand every word, the techniques used or even the results. In fact, I can almost guarantee that you will not. At the beginning, I even read a few theses that were outside my scope of practice, from oncology to rowing biomechanics. At this point, it is not about gaining detail on the specifics; it is about getting a general overview of what a thesis is and looks like, so that it becomes less scary and more of an inspiration to begin writing and even thinking about the layout of your work. At the beginning be curious, enjoy and feel free to explore.

Start Writing Early

When I began my doctorate, several experienced academics advised me to begin writing early. Writing seemed like a fool's errand in the early days, as I had no data, let alone results. However, don't let this discourage you. There is a lot you can begin with, even in early stages. In fact, a lot of the work that I did at this point really helped me at the end, when I had more time pressure and detailed writing to undertake.

In my first year of doctoral studies, I attended a course led by the university about how to lay out my thesis in a format that was acceptable to the university. Each university will have free courses that are available to you in this regard, and it's a great way of getting to know the accepted format. It's really important to become familiar with the university regulations early on and to keep abreast of any changes. It was at such a course that I learned key tips in terms of thesis layout, expectations, formal paperwork required, rules and regulations in relation to plagiarism and other such topics. If such a course is available at your university or you can meet with someone to discuss these elements further, then I recommend it. Put simply, it is always better to know what the expectations are well in advance so that you are well prepared from the beginning. Although most of the information related to thesis writing is usually housed on the university website, attending this course enabled me to meet fellow doctoral students, some of whom are still friends to this day. It also helped me to put a face to the names of the key university administrative team members, which helped when it came to requesting administrative support.

Thesis requirements vary between universities. In an effort to share with you what this general format may look like, a typical thesis skeleton usually consists of an introduction, methodology, results, discussion and conclusions. In this respect, it is almost like a very large scientific paper. However, how you write it will depend entirely on your research. So, for example, your research may focus on one specific area, in which case your thesis may be represented as an entire story from beginning to end. However, if you use mixed methods and have a few very different smaller studies to discuss, each chapter may require its own introduction, methodology, results, discussion and conclusions.

My research involved many different methods and protocols, so each of my studies had results that required critical discussion and conclusions. The final chapter included a summary discussion and conclusions section that tied up the threads from each chapter so that complex findings arising from individual biomechanical patient studies became easier to interpret.

Theses may be written 'by publication' or not. This is dependent on the university requirements, so again, it will be necessary for you to check this locally. Thesis by publication means that your thesis is presented as a collection of papers that you have written throughout the doctorate. In some ways, this makes sense as it means that the vast majority of your publications are then finished by the time you submit your thesis. In my case, the university specified that thesis by publication was not permitted; however, I was able to add any open access papers within the appendix. Therefore, I cannot emphasise how vital it is to check university regulations in advance to guide your approach.

Writing Wins

Quick wins are extremely important in enhancing your motivation to write your thesis. During the thesis-writing phase, I recall hitting the proverbial brick wall. It did not matter what I did; I could not move forward. I relayed the experience to a colleague in the same position, and she said kindly, 'Remember there is always something you can do with a thesis.' To this day I have never forgotten these words. You will have great writing days and days that are not so great in terms of word count, but it is important to remember that whatever day you are having, there is always something you can do.

Quick wins, to me, are the things that you can do to motivate you, to feel that you are moving positively in the right direction. These quick wins can be as you define them. In terms of a thesis, there will always be a protocol to write, a graph that you can design, a spell check that you can perform, references that require refining. Although you may not be up for a big day of writing or may feel as if you have little to write, there is always something you can do to help you feel as if you are winning.

Mind Mapping

At the beginning of my thesis, my first quick win was simply a mind map of what it would look like. I love to draw and am quite a visual learner, so for me, mapping it out really helped. This map was a unique overview of my plan, a chance to present my thesis in my way. I was first introduced to the idea of mind mapping by one of the best clinical educators I ever had. He introduced me to the author Tony Buzan and showed me how powerful mind mapping could be in developing patterns of thought and creating order from disorder.

When undertaking a doctorate, there is so much to learn and there are so many possibilities that there is a definite need to create more order. I slowly found that through the overwhelming effect of many texts, publications and ideas, regular engagement with my doctoral mind map could help to crystallise my thoughts. It was a map that could evolve as my ideas matured, and as they did, there was a place in my notebook for them. For me the ideas came more easily when I wrote them and drew them within my favourite notebook. Somehow it felt freer this way, as it was not a computer screen, where there is a temptation to self-edit and become critical as one writes. Like an artist at an easel, I was able to create without judgement, which made the process fun. Sometimes I really got into it and would wake first thing in the morning when my head was filled with ideas, make a hot cup of English Breakfast tea, and when the house was quiet and the world had not awoken yet, I would draw and write. Doing this in a way that is special for you is important, as writing is such an integral part of becoming a researcher that enjoying the process and making it work for you are half the battle.

How you structure your first mind map is totally up to you. My first one looked like a spaghetti junction of thoughts and reworked ideas, which I slowly refined. However, I found it useful to create a central bubble in which I placed a provisional title with my principal research question, hypothesis, aims and objectives. From this, like spokes of a wheel, I began to plot the provisional titles for each chapter in separate bubbles. I also included bubbles for appendices and references to begin to think about how these might look and what they might contain.

This process can look or feel however you wish. You may prefer to create a mood board of thoughts as a poster or create a mind map using Padlet or similar online software. Whatever way you choose, it is important to work in the way that you work best and in which ideas flow for you without restriction. This great quick win can then be used to create your first doctoral thesis template and is useful to return to when you feel you are losing your focus or need to get into your helicopter to see the overarching picture. Don't be afraid to update it and amend it. In fact, by retaining your mind map history, you can document your journey and use the maps to affirm just how far you have come.

Document as You Go

Although mind maps are a great way of visualising progress and getting an overview of where you are headed, it is also useful to document your way. When you are on your thesis-writing mission, you will at times forget why you made the decisions you did and the limitations you experienced. However, it is important to remember your rationale and specific details from your unique experience to support your writing and viva defence.

Some days ideas will simply pop into your head that will inform your thesis or inform future work. When this happens, all I can say is document, document, document. I used an ideas folder on my desktop, which I added to as these ideas cropped up. My research supervisor recommended this, and it is a technique that I use to this day. Although you may not use every idea you have, it can be useful for future planning and future work. I also used my most favourite notebook to document experiences and reasoning that related to the specific chapters I had previously outlined in my mind map. You may even find it useful to have a notebook at your bedside so that when ideas or reflections come, you can add them to the page and get them out of your head, or you can use your mobile phone to record notes as you go. Of course, there are many ways of doing this. One of my friends found voice recording software useful so that she could talk and walk through her ideas. The most important thing is to go with your gut instinct on this. Do what works for you.

I found documenting my ideas particularly helpful in my final year, as ideas were coming thick and fast. By committing ideas to paper they no longer occupy your head, which is particularly helpful when the thoughts become invasive—and they do. The way this showed up for me included difficulty in being completely present in important everyday activities. My husband would often accuse me of daydreaming. I remember I used to laugh at this ,but he was right. I believe my brain was so filled with new ideas and reflections that it became difficult to focus on anything else. While this is understandable towards the final few months of thesis writing, when your focus deserves and needs to be on your sleep or clinical work or being with your family, it becomes a really important practice to document your thoughts, rendering your brain free and capable fulfilling important commitments outside of your doctorate.

Bite-Sized Writing

As a parent, doctoral student and clinician, you quickly learn that every minute of the day counts, and you become very efficient in the way you use your time. Bite-sized writing, as I call it, really helped me to feel that I was making progress at every stage of my doctoral journey. Bite-sized writing means that you write as you are able. For healthcare professionals, it is not easy to write a thesis alongside professional work commitments, and this does not even take into account additional personal commitments.

Although I discuss writing in more detail in Chapter 9, if we focus on bite-sized writing as it applies specifically to a thesis, this could mean writing up your research protocols or methods as you go. In general, the process of writing up protocols or research methods is straightforward and can really make you feel as if you are winning. I found it easiest to set up a template for each chapter according to the layout requirements of the university. The template could then be populated and revised as I had the time and inclination.

On the basis that there is always something you can do with a thesis, the first bite-sized writing step I took was to set my title page and chapter headers according to my original mind map. This will change and be revised as you go, but this is OK. Just starting from something that looks less like a blank page and more like a thesis will really help you. As you begin populating your template and house all related information in one place, the document will become a launchpad from which abstracts and papers may be written. Conversely, if you write a paper or an abstract for a conference first, you may use these ideas to populate your thesis. It will be important that you do not self-plagiarise in this instance, so seek plagiarism guidance from your university to make sure that you are following best writing practice.

In terms of the thesis writing order, people adopt different methods. However, for me, I found it best to write the methods section first. Once I processed and analysed my data, I then wrote the results section. From there I felt prepared to write the discussion and conclusions. Finally, and perhaps counterintuitively, I wrote the introduction and abstract. Although I always thought that it would be important to write the thesis in order (introduction first, followed by methods, results, discussion and conclusions), this is not always the case. In fact, I found it easier to write and hone the introduction and abstract for the chapter after I had written the results and could appreciate the conclusions.

Reframing Writing

As you make progress writing your thesis, you may notice that you tire of it. This is why it becomes so important that you reframe the process. What would writing look like to you if it were fun? Would there be music? Would writing a section of your thesis alongside friends help? Do you need a change of venue? It is really important to have what you need on the day when thesis writing becomes a seemingly tiresome activity.

When I was writing my thesis, there were times when I would listen to free online music playlists that were said to increase writing productivity and focus. Sometimes I would work in environments that I knew increased my productivity, such as the library, or I would try to create such an environment at home when I could not get to the library because of competing demands on my time. I recall that one day when I needed to write and the environment was not working for me, I searched for 'library sounds' and found that those exact sounds were freely available on line. It seems almost unimaginable that you can find something so specific, but you can. If you know you need the sound of the rain to make you feel calm or alpha waves to focus your mind, search for them and use them to reframe your writing practice. Equally, if you write better with a focussed screen, turn notification off and use a focussed display on your computer or a writing lamp to improve your focus and productivity.

Writing your thesis in your way is all about knowing how you write best. Reflect on days when you have had a positive thesis-writing experience, days when your writing just flowed. What did they look like and how could you re-create them? Often, you will realise that you don't need anything fancy or expensive or even to go anywhere special. Sometimes you can re-create these writing experiences by simply altering the sounds you experience, the light, the community you surround yourself with or not. Do it your way!

Be Organised and Back It Up!

If you wish to win at writing your thesis it is key that you are organised and that you regularly save and back up your work. In my experience, I found it useful to assign a version number, name and date to each chapter draft. This helps when sharing documents for feedback purposes, and also, if you ever delete a version in error, you may return to the original file without a problem. For this reason, at each writing session, I would create and save a new version of the chapter I was working on. All I can advise is never to delete the versions you have created. You never know when you will need them.

Although it is out of the scope of this chapter to comment exactly on how to back up your work, it is extremely important to do so regularly, automatically if possible, and to discuss any queries with the information technology specialist at your university. At the time I undertook my doctorate, I was encouraged to save copies on an external drive, on my university computer, and within the university cloud. I was also advised to house copies of my external hard drive at different locations so that if a fire took hold in a laboratory or a hard drive was stolen from my home, it would not be a problem. Although the advice may change with time, in my opinion, you cannot be overcautious. By planning your backup measures and consulting the right people in advance, you will avoid unnecessary heartache.

Writing by Publication

In some cases, a thesis may be submitted by publication. This means that the thesis contains a set of papers and each publication forms a chapter within the thesis. This is very different from a traditional thesis, which is not a collection of papers. Instead, a traditional thesis contains unpublished work (introduction, methods, results, discussion and conclusions) and may reference papers published during the doctoral process within the appendix.

Since there is such a distinction between 'thesis by publication' and a traditional approach, I encourage you to seek advice at the earliest opportunity from your supervisors and the university so that you may be assured that you are following the correct standards.

If your thesis is by publication, then it is usually important to have your manuscripts submitted and published before submitting your final thesis. If you are intending to submit your work for publication, here are a few simple considerations that you may find helpful:

- When publishing your work, consider the scope of the journal that you are planning to submit to. The scope is usually available on the website. If your research is outside the scope of the journal, it is unlikely that it will be published.
- If you are unsure which journals to submit to, ask your supervisors, and take a look at journals that have previously published work similar to yours.
- Carefully review the journal author information for specific guidance in terms of accepted layout and terms and conditions of publication. Again, if you do not consider the specifics, you are unlikely to be successful.
- Before submitting your article, remember that all co-authors need to review the article and approve its submission. If this is not the case, the article will not be published.
- Consider open access journals, as this may mean that you will be able to republish an article as part of your thesis without fear of plagiarism. However, open access publication requires funding, so it will be important to understand the journals your university supports in this regard.
- If the manuscript is accepted, the editor will advise you as to how to proceed. However, if minor or major changes are required, you will be notified and will receive detailed feedback from the editor, which you will be expected to respond to on a point by point basis. It is important to deal with each comment in a respectful and reasoned manner so that the reviewer is assured that you have dealt with any issues, or that if you disagree with the comments provided, there is a reasonable suggestion offered as to why this was the case.
- If the submitted manuscript is rejected, don't worry. This happens to the best of us and is an important part of your research journey. If rejected, remember to ask for feedback, if this has not already been provided. In this way you will be able to move forward and to address any modifiable features. Remember to consult with your team, including your doctoral supervisors, regarding next steps. Usually these will involve submitting your work to another journal. The existing manuscript may require reformatting in order to make this possible. Review the author information for the new journal you have selected, as the guidance varies between journals. In some cases, the editor may ask you if you would like them to export your article directly to another journal of theirs that they think may be more appropriate, in which case there will be few if any changes required.
- Avoid scams or phishing e-mails that encourage you to publish your work with an unknown publisher. Scam e-mails will often address you as 'Dr' or 'Professor' even though you are not, are usually from an unknown journal or one unrelated to your area of work and advise you to click a link to upload your work. The problem here is that if you upload your work, you do not know where it is going, how it will be used and by whom, and there is nearly always an associated publication cost. If you receive such e-mails, consult your information technology department or your supervisor to double check. Be safe!

Feedback Is Your Friend

The thought of receiving feedback is often terrifying when you begin a doctorate. Will you meet the mark? Is your work good enough to meet the doctoral standard? Somehow when you begin a doctorate it is often a temptation to apply a perfectionist approach, meaning that before we let it go for feedback, we take care to go through everything in infinitesimal detail, and even then it does not feel good enough. However, I need to encourage you to let go of your thesis writing early so that you can receive feedback sooner rather than later. If you are not taking the right approach, it is really important to find this out early.

I remember that when I had written my first doctoral abstract for a conference I was terrified to let it go and to receive feedback. During the first few months of my doctorate, I knew I had good work to share with the world, but I was scared to let it go. I remember phoning my father, who always provided the best counsel. He said, 'Think of the worst case scenario; then if you are OK with the worst case, it will be OK'. My worst case scenario was to receive hurtful comments from my supervisors. However, knowing my supervisors, I knew that any comments would be sent with the intention of advancing and improving my work. So why would I not want this? It would be OK. Now as I sit here as a supervisor of doctoral students, I know this to be true. We want the best for all of our students, and therefore, we try to communicate our feedback in a constructive and respectful manner.

Letting go of your thesis chapters for feedback is sometimes difficult, as they become almost part of you when you write them. From Elizabeth Gilbert, I have understood that some authors think about their novels as their babies, in that they were lovingly created, nurtured and birthed when they were published. I must admit that I although I never quite thought of my thesis in this way, I can see how this attachment can occur when you are simply eating, sleeping and breathing the words you are writing. Perhaps this attachment is why it is hard to let go of your thesis for review? However, it is important to submit draft sections of your thesis for feedback as soon as you can. It is a necessary part of understanding where you are and whether further support and direction are required. So don't worry about it being perfect, let alone about birthing it; once it is in a 'good enough' state, just let it go.

Feedback and Knowing What You Need

When asking for feedback on your thesis, it is really important that you know what feedback you need. Doctoral supervisors are busy people, so if you wish to receive prompt and relevant feedback, it is important to be specific. So, for example, if you are writing an e-mail you might identify two or three bullet points that you would like them to cover. These bullet points could include questions such as 'Is the title clear?' 'Are my results presented succinctly enough?' or 'My conclusion indicates x, is this correct?'. This will greatly help your supervisors. It is also useful to provide a deadline by which you would like to receive feedback, particularly if this relates to something that is time sensitive. Be advised that the depth of the feedback you receive will usually correspond to the amount of time that you give your supervisors to offer comment, so try not to send documents at the last minute. This will never yield the best results.

Sometimes there is a temptation to ask for more feedback than you require in order to build your confidence. You may ask for feedback from many peers, colleagues, supervisors or experts in the area in order to validate your work. However, it is really important that feedback is focussed. It needs to be provided by the most appropriate people. Before taking a scattergun approach, consider not only why and when you require feedback but also from whom. There is nothing more unsettling than receiving feedback from too many people. They will all have a different focus and bias. Therefore, this approach often serves to confuse and unsettle you and may even act as a roadblock as you try to satisfy them. Know that you can never satisfy everyone and that this is not your job. Your job is to seek feedback in a timely manner from the right people and to use this to move your research forward. Be guided by your instinct, your opinion and direction. Remember you are the expert on what you need.

Dealing With Feedback

Feedback may be provided internally by your supervisors, mentors or peers or externally by examiners or journal reviewers. Sometimes feedback may be difficult to take, particularly if it is not complimentary, and I think as a doctoral student you need to be open to this possibility. As you grow as a researcher, you will realise that the world will not always agree with you or your ideas, and that this is OK. People will have different opinions and may not always be kind in the way that they express this. For example, when submitting articles for journal publication or sample chapters to your supervisors, often you will receive feedback that you may not agree with, or you may not appreciate the way in which the feedback is expressed. Sometimes the feedback can be quite direct and may appear unkind in some cases. When you are in the early stages of a research career, it is difficult not to take this personally, but it is important that you don't. Often feedback is written by busy researchers who may not have had the time to review their comments or may not appreciate the way in which their words come across. Therefore, you may find it useful to create some distance between you and the feedback.

There are many ways to create distance. First, after you read the feedback, it may be useful to take a day where you step away from the feedback and consider the big picture: What are they trying to tell you? what elements are they suggesting that could make your article better? if you addressed the comments, would it enhance your article? Since the answer to the latter is often 'yes', then following your break from the feedback you will feel in a better place to deal with it. Second, once you have taken a break from the feedback, it will be important to read the feedback again in more detail. Think about what they are saying to you. Take each point and remove what is subjective from the comments. By making the feedback more objective, you can create action points to deal with each comment. So for example, a comment such as 'This title is totally confusing, nobody will be able to understand this!' might become 'Title needs to be clear'. Suddenly, you have taken a comment that appears hopeless and converted it into something that is actionable and positive. It is important to remember that reviewers are human, and as humans, communication may not always be so well considered. Keep this in mind when you read any feedback and do not let it affect you negatively; rather, turn it around and make it count. Make it actionable and *for* you rather than *against* you.

Thesis Requirements

The thesis is your own account of your research, and in this respect it is very important that you take ownership and accountability for everything that is stated within it. The thesis should make a distinct, original contribution to your field in that it represents new information that has not previously been discovered. It should present a cohesive story so that all the threads are linked and a rational argument is provided. This will require a depth of knowledge, criticality and research skill that will need to be demonstrated within the thesis. The thesis requirements will be determined by the university that you are attending. It will be critical that you are aware of what the requirements are in order to meet them. Requirements may also change during the period of your doctorate, so it will be important to keep updated.

The doctoral thesis requirements are usually outlined clearly by each university in terms of how the thesis should be presented and written, including the word count. To give you an idea of what a word count might be like for a doctoral thesis, my university specified that the word count should not exceed 100,000 words. I found this word count to be entirely reasonable, in that there was enough freedom to be able to express my ideas and discoveries and yet the word count discouraged the potential lack of focus that could have been incurred by writing above 100,000 words.

The thesis requirements should also include regulations regarding examination misconduct. At my university misconduct included but was not limited to (1) false representation of the work of others, (2) fabrication of data, and (3) submission of research commissioned from another individual. In addition, allegations of plagiarism will also be considered as an examination offence. Theses will usually be examined for plagiarism by the external examiners and using additional plagiarism software. If you wish to become aware of the policies and procedures regarding examination offences, it will be important to review the university website or to consult your academic registrar directly. Universities take examination misconduct very seriously, so please ensure that you take steps to align with the policies and procedures at your university.

Thesis Submission

Thesis submission deadlines are usually set by the university. Submission deadlines are set to ensure parity between students and will vary depending on the way you are undertaking your doctorate (part time or full time). It is a requirement to meet this deadline to ensure that your doctoral award is granted. If you hold an external grant, funding bodies will expect you to meet this deadline. However, some may experience difficulties around the time of submission. This may include unpredictable events such as family bereavement or illness, in which case your supervisor will guide you as to how to apply for an extension to alleviate the pressure on you at such an important time in the process. It is key to contact your supervisors as soon as you know you are having difficulties so that they may support you in the best way. Indeed, regular communication really helps at times like this, so that everyone is updated. If you require further assistance, there are also student support services or disability teams that may assist if reasonable adjustments need to be put in place. Reasonable adjustments could include changes to the examination conditions (when and where it occurs or the time you have to undertake an exam) or changes to the submission deadline.

In terms of submission requirements, some academic institutions will request the submission of an electronic and/or paper copy of the thesis. However, for some, as in my case, it was purely an electronic submission process. Therefore, it is recommended that you become aware of the preferred practice at your university so that you can ensure that everything is delivered on time and in the right format. The deadlines for submission are usually strict, so it is important that this is met. Doing this is really all about preparation.

Before submission, it is a good idea to have people read your thesis or thesis chapters. Some students will choose to pay for external editors to review their theses. Colleagues and friends of mine used this method, as they were under time pressure. However, in my opinion, this is an expensive option and is not necessary. If you have time and have planned well, your examiners will have reviewed your entire thesis before submission, and you will have also read it thoroughly. I even asked some of my family to read it; you would be surprised what they picked up. In this way, you can avoid unnecessary costs and feel assured that the work you are submitting is of high quality.

In advance of the final submission deadline, it is important to plan. This may include thinking about additional childcare for the final weeks before your deadline or taking annual leave to give you more space and time. Some of my colleagues even asked friends to cook for them during the final month. The time before thesis submission is critical, is intense and requires pure focus, so this is the time to call in all your favours, to gain support from wherever you can and submerge yourself in the final preparation.

My final thesis submission deadline was set by the university in the first year of my doctorate. However, despite this, my husband and I decided that I needed to submit earlier. Although I had set the expectations for my final doctoral year in advance, in the end it was becoming too difficult for my husband to be a single parent to two toddlers in the final months, and I missed them. Therefore, doing my PhD my way meant I needed to respect the needs of my entire family and submit early.

I must admit that submitting before the deadline is not for the faint-hearted, but for me, my family is the most important thing in my life. Therefore, I needed to listen to them and compromise. I am sharing this as I feel it's important to know that there can be flexibility depending on your personal requirements, and so in discussion with my supervisors I submitted early. This required a lot of late nights and early mornings, caffeination and becoming a frequent visitor of libraries and coffee shops, or anywhere I could find peace and quiet. Relative consistency was required and during this time I elected to eat, sleep and dream my thesis. In the later stages this felt like the best way forward.

Enjoy Your Final Day

I will never forget the final day of writing my thesis. On that cold December day, I asked my husband if I could use his quiet office space. There was snow everywhere and the heating was barely working in the office. I wore layers of jumpers and wrapped myself with my large scarf, which was with me from the very beginning of the journey. In honour of the preparatory writing ritual to which I had become accustomed during my doctorate, I made a hot cup of breakfast tea as I watched the snow fall outside the window. Although I did not tell my husband or any of my family or friends, I knew that this was the day. This was the day I would submit.

On that day, I used the time to read lovingly through the pages of what seemed to be my life for the past few years. As I read, it was a trip down memory lane. I remembered each person who had helped me along the way, the patients, the students, mentors, supervisors and researchers. I recalled the hours it took to make bespoke pieces of equipment with engineering colleagues to enable certain research projects, the fun I had creating a marker set to evaluate patient movement, the frustration when a specific programming script would not run because line 153 had an error in it. In that moment, I could sit back and enjoy it all.

Once I had lovingly completed the final read-through, I returned to the beginning of my thesis to read the acknowledgements and my dedication to the people who mattered to me: my teachers, my patients, my family. I read it and predictably cried my last tears. I had succeeded in writing my thesis and was proud. I entered the university web platform for doctorate submission and pressed Submit. There was no going back. I had done it.

Although online thesis submission can feel a little underwhelming, I decided to personalise this day and to mark the occasion. That evening I pretended to my children and husband that I needed to go to a local village to collect some books, when, in fact, I had booked a table for four at a beautiful little restaurant. Once we entered the restaurant, we were guided to a comfortable nook for four that was surrounded by paintings of local wildlife and flowers. While my boys gazed at the menu in awe, I secretly ordered champagne. In the same moment that the chilled, elegant overflowing glasses were delivered to the table, I announced that I had submitted my thesis and that it was all over. My husband was overjoyed, and I think my sons were too. However, for my boys, it was possibly the prospect of having chocolate pudding for dessert that excited them more. Therefore, when all is said and done and your thesis is submitted, I encourage you too to celebrate with those who have made it all possible. You simply cannot do it without them.

Finding Your Way: Thesis Writing — Learning Points

- You will never feel 'ready' to write a thesis, so just write.
- Theses are available to read at online university portals, and hard copies may also be available. Review theses in and outside your scope of practice to understand the expectations.
- Begin writing early. This can include simply writing up methods sections or protocols to begin with, or setting up a working thesis template.
- Consider using a mind map to develop an overview of your thesis plan and to encourage focus.
- Remember to document as you go so that you remember all of the steps you took on your journey. This could include any changes in your protocols, limitations you experienced or revisions.
- Bite-sized thesis writing will help to motivate you on a day when time is limited. Remember there is always something you can do with a thesis!
- Reframe your thesis writing on difficult writing days. Consider what you need to get into a writing flow (music, change of environment, community).
- Save and back up your work regularly. Seek advice from information technology specialists from your university to avoid problems.
- Ask for feedback from supervisors, friends and experts as you require it. Remember to be specific with your request. What do you want feedback on? When do you need feedback by? Be clear.
- Be aware of the university thesis requirements and keep updated. This will be your responsibility.
- Plan for your thesis submission in advance. Organise the support and time you need to meet your submission deadline.
- Acknowledge those who have supported your doctoral experience and celebrate your submission.

Finding Your Way: Thesis Writing — Action Points

The most important action points that I can act on today/this week/this month are

Finding Your Way: Thesis Writing — Steps Towards Achieving Action Points

The next steps I can take towards these action points are

_____
_____
_____
_____
_____
_____
_____
_____
_____
_____
_____
_____
_____
_____
_____
_____
_____
_____
_____
_____
_____
_____
_____
_____
_____
_____
_____
_____
_____
_____
_____
_____
_____
_____
_____
_____
_____
_____
_____
_____
_____
_____

CHAPTER 11

Viva Voce

I come as one but I stand as ten thousand.
—Maya Angelou

Viva voce is a Latin phrase meaning 'with living voice'. It is commonly termed the 'viva' and is a way in which doctoral students are examined following completion of their doctoral research and submission of their thesis. As an assessment, the viva is designed to give students space and time to discuss their unique research contribution with experts in the area. In the United Kingdom, the examining team usually consists of internal and external examiners selected by the university. However, in some countries, university staff, family and the general public may also be invited to attend the doctoral viva.

At the beginning of one's research journey, it is usual to feel that the viva is an insurmountable hill to climb. At least this was my feeling at the very beginning of my doctorate. However, I have found from my experience as an educator, clinician and researcher that, at the end of the process, there is simply nothing better than having the opportunity to share your research absolutely and completely with people who are interested in your work. At the end of your doctoral journey, it is quite simply a gift to be able to communicate your journey in your way.

Viva Preparation

When I undertook my doctorate, I was required to submit written reports and present research updates as part of a university doctoral review process. This milestone review process was designed to ensure that the work was of sufficient quality and met doctoral requirements. While this may look different at different universities, it is important to embrace any opportunity to present and share your work. In the end, it is such opportunities that will prepare you in the best way for your viva and ultimately your future research career, where the defence and dissemination of your work become important.

In preparation for your viva and for your subsequent career in research, it is important to share your research in different ways: to present at national and international conferences, to discuss your research with key stakeholders (patients, clinicians, managers), to network, to join committees and to communicate your research to different audiences. It is these experiences that help to build the confidence required to defend your research, to communicate your unique contribution succinctly and to provide a rationale for your work. By sowing these seeds from the beginning of the doctoral process, you are paving the way for a positive viva experience.

Discussion With Peers

Looking back, my preparation for the viva began from the very start of my doctoral studies. This was largely because I didn't ever feel I could take this opportunity for granted. It was important to me, to my patients and to clinicians who came after me that I get it right. I think this is true for most clinical researchers. The gravity of the responsibility we hold for our patients, hospitals, colleagues and funders is real, as we are often doing something that has not been done before within our profession.

For me to prepare for my viva, I decided that it was important to discuss the viva experience with clinicians and academics who had succeeded in this process. As is my character, I asked them every question I could think of in order to feel more confident on the day. Successful post-doctoral researchers kindly shared their amazing viva stories with me. The stories were varied and extreme. For most the experience was really uplifting, with people recollecting the welcome and liberating closure associated with the viva experience. However, for some, the experience was challenging. In these cases, challenges usually related to issues during the doctoral process that remained unre-solved, including funding issues, inadequate doctoral support or problems with the supervisory relationship. While it is important to consider both sides, it can be difficult to envision a positive outcome if you dwell too deeply upon the negative experiences of others.

Therefore, as part of your preparatory journey, I suggest bathing yourself in optimism so that you believe success is possible for you as you swim towards it. Indeed, to reinforce a positive per-spective, supervisors often advise you to remember that you are the expert on your own research. Although this is something that I did not quite believe, it was always empowering to consider this possibility. Having circumnavigated all obstacles and undertaken your research independently, feel assured that your supervisors are correct: nobody understands your research better than you. On the day of your viva, you will be the expert.

Viva Plan

As my viva beckoned, I tried to identify the key aspects of viva success. Everyone I talked to had a different perspective, which I would later understand was their way. However, to find mine, I needed to embrace these experiences and find out what would work best for me. Dur-ing this time peers shared some interesting ideas, including what to wear and what snacks to bring. The consideration of such specifics become key on the day of the viva, since the viva examination can take anything from one to nine hours depending on the university, supervi-sors and student requirements. This means that you may be sitting for a prolonged period dur-ing intense discussions. If you are wearing uncomfortable clothes or are hungry, for example, it will be difficult to perform well. Therefore, it is really important to consider your specific needs and to plan well.

There is no 'one size fits all' plan to prepare for your viva. However, I would like to share some ideas that you may find helpful. First, know your examiners. Examiners are usually selected based upon their particular research expertise, which usually aligns with the research undertaken by the doctoral student. It is usual for the lead university supervisor to facilitate examiner selection and to extend an invitation to each examiner at a date and time that is convenient for both you and them. Take time to review the research profiles and publications of your examiners in advance of your viva. This will increase your confidence and ensure that your discussions may be more meaningful and that your exchanges respect each other's professional viewpoints. For example, the way you discuss your thesis with a professor of physiology may be very different from the slant you may take with a professor of biomechanics.

Second, know your location. Where will your viva take place? Will it be in an auditorium or a room? How many will be in attendance? Will you be seated opposite your examiners? Will they be examining you from a different location via a virtual platform? Simple things such as visiting the room where your viva will take place and thinking about how you might like the furniture arranged (if this is possible) can help. This may seem crazy. However, for some, having a table between the student and examiners can elevate performance, while for others, it may prove intimidating, in which case, having no table and a circle of chairs with sufficient personal space is better. This is why knowing yourself and your way is so important to your performance on the day.

Don't be afraid to ask for what you need. I have found that any reasonable requests are generally well received.

Knowing the location, room setup and who would be in attendance on the day of my viva really helped in terms of planning and visualisation. As with athletes, visualisation and mental rehearsal can be extremely useful for doctoral students. Imagining what success on the day feels like and looks like, visualising yourself in the room, thinking of what you might say, your delight and the excitement of your family and friends when you share the news of your success, visualising who you will become and how this could change future outcomes for your patients may all be used to prepare and enhance your viva performance.

Reasonable Adjustments

If you have a disability or require any specific additional support, it is possible for reasonable adjustments to be made. Most universities have disability support services that can put important adjustments in place well in advance of the viva, and this can be done in liaison with your supervisors. How this happens will vary and will be dependent on the university that you attend. However, it will be important to be proactive—to ask the questions you need to and plan in advance. It is my belief that every student deserves to feel comfortable and capable of performing confidently and without compromise. In this respect, universities and supervisors are happy to support anything that will optimise your confidence and performance.

Tips for Viva Day

With all of this in mind, here are some additional quick tips that you may wish to consider in preparation for viva day:

1. The viva can be a lengthy process, so make sure you bring along some supplies just in case you are hungry or thirsty (e.g., water and simple snacks such as nuts or a banana).
2. Wear comfortable clothes that inspire you to perform with confidence. If you are unsure of the dress code, simply ask your supervisor.
3. Make sure that you have plenty of time to get to the venue. I had several travel plans (train, bus, taxi) in case there were travel problems on the day.
4. Bring along a phone and computer charger. A phone is essential, particularly to share the good news of your success with your family at the end of the day!
5. It is useful to have a copy of your thesis in your bag. If your mind goes blank or you wish to refer to a specific graph, having a copy of your thesis (paper or electronic) may support you with recall and help you to relax.
6. There is no 'right way' here, so just think about what you need to support yourself in advance and do that.

Sticky Notes and Highlights

On the day of the viva, I found that my thesis was, surprisingly, one of the most important tools. I never realised that this would be the case until one weekend I visited a friend of mine who had recently completed her viva. Her file- and paper-filled study, with a jungle of books and stationery on the floor, was so familiar to me. Although it seemed chaotic, there was a definite order to the way in which her papers were organised. Amongst it all, her thesis stood proudly, well-thumbed and adorned with sticky notes.

At the time, I was curious to see a thesis for the first time, to understand the expectations that lay ahead of me. I asked her permission to leaf through the well-crafted, precious pages. When I held that book, I could appreciate the hours and the effort that went into creating it. I could almost feel the perspiration, the tears and the joy that went into each chapter. However, more curiously, I was drawn to the bright markings in each chapter, the sticky squares of coloured paper that were filled with notes and the underlined phrases and key words that lay within.

I would later adopt the same approach with my thesis. I learned that by using coloured index flags I could quickly locate relevant chapters. Since it is customary for examiners to discuss any chapter in any order, using these flags meant that I could identify the chapter during the viva and if they referred to a diagram or table, I could easily locate it and refer to it directly. I also found it useful to underline key lines of text and used sticky notes to house some keyword reminders that I thought might slip my mind if I was anxious. As I have always liked real books rather than e-books and love stationery, it seemed perfectly natural for me to work with a paper copy of my thesis. I certainly found that organising my thesis in this way not only helped with viva preparation but also helped to reduce my anxiety and to increase my feeling of control of the day. However, it is perfectly possible to use the same approach using an electronic copy of your thesis. Again, it is as you define it. Go with what works for you.

Organise a Practice Viva

In preparation for the day, some find it useful to organise a practice viva. It is usual for this to be arranged with your supervisors or members of your team who have experience in undertaking vivas at this level. Usually, students plan for practice vivas to occur between the submission of their thesis and the viva itself. Whatever timeline you choose, it is key to give yourself enough time to reflect upon your feedback. If you plan your practice viva too close to the actual day of the viva, it may derail you if the feedback you receive is not 100% positive or affirming. Remember that a practice viva is an optional activity and does not form part of the formal viva process.

My lead supervisor kindly offered me the possibility of a practice viva. However, I felt that this was not something I required, and it is important to know that this is also an option. I felt assured through consistent presentation of my work and feedback provided by my university that I was ready. For me, I just needed time to simply 'be' before my viva. At the time, my grandmother had just died and with two young children, I needed time: time to relax, to visualise success, to read my thesis and to be calm. Due to my particular circumstances, I did not need the pressure of another event to prepare for. For me, the preparation began long before this time. I had presented my research at many national and international conferences, I had discussed and shared my research across professions and in different ways and had published my work. Doing the viva my way meant having absolutely and completely what I needed. This involved a quiet and contemplative preparation period. I chose to exercise and meditate quietly every day, to nourish my body with healthy food, to read my thesis and to spend quiet time with my family. I felt confident and assured that my work was done and that all of the preparation from the beginning of my doctorate had led to this day. Preparation from the beginning gave me this time. If you are in a similar position, discuss your plan with your supervisors and feel encouraged to do what you feel is best for you.

You Are Not Alone

It may sound strange to say this, but on the day of my viva, I did not feel that I walked alone. Yes, it was me who submitted the thesis, and yes, it was me sitting there in front of a panel of examiners. However, as Professor Maya Angelou describes, we are never truly alone. You may come as one, but you can stand as ten thousand in any room when you are surrounded by all of those who have preceded you or made your journey possible. I found this quite an empowering thought. As the first in my family to enter a doctoral viva, I did as Professor Angelou described: I visualised my entire family behind me, the researchers and clinicians who had trailblazed the path, the funders and patients, all of whom made it possible for me to accept this privilege. They were all there.

The Viva Process

It is important to become acquainted with the viva protocol in your university and the criteria by which you will be marked on the day. Although the viva process may vary between universities, I would like to share my viva experience with you. Before I undertook my viva, it was necessary to submit an electronic copy to the university (some universities may also require a paper copy). The university then distributed my thesis to my respective examiners for review in advance of the viva. This gives examiners time to read the thesis in more detail, to grade it in line with the university criteria and to think of questions that they would like to pose on the day. There is usually a marking system adopted by each university to ensure that all students are marked in a similar way, and both internal and external examiners ensure that this is the case.

On the viva day, once you are seated and comfortable, it is customary for the examiners to explain how the process will run from beginning to end. In my case, this included introducing basic ground rules, when I could expect breaks, who would ask questions first and when I would receive notification of the outcome. The examiners then usually begin with questions to help orient you and make you feel welcome. The first few questions are designed to relax you and to make you feel at ease. So, for me, the first examiner asked me to briefly describe my research, including my research question, why my research was important and why it made a unique contribution. Doctorates are awarded for novel work, and part of your job is to demonstrate the unique contribution that your research will make. As mentioned, it is beneficial to review the specific criteria that the examiners will use to grade you. However, here are some of the typical criteria that may be used to evaluate doctoral work:

- the work represents the genuine work of the candidate;
- it makes a distinct contribution to knowledge in this area;
- it is original, demonstrating critical power and discovery of new facts;
- it is of a standard to merit publication.

During the viva, it is quite normal to experience moments where you forget a figure or a name or something relevant to the discussion. In this situation, it is important to be kind to yourself, to take your time and to remember that examiners are willing for you to succeed. You may also find it useful to consider some of the following suggestions if you are having difficulty understanding a question or your memory is not serving you well:

- If you have not understood a question or could not hear it, it is OK to ask the examiner to repeat it.
- If you cannot answer the question because you need time to consider the answer, it is OK to ask for time and to come back to this question later.
- If you do not know the answer to the question, it is OK to say, 'I do not know,' and to relate to another similar case in point, or to ask for their opinion on this area so that you may learn. Remember that this is a professional discussion and that as human beings we do not always know the answer to everything.

However, a note of caution. It is important to remember that the above suggestions are to be used sparingly and only in exceptional circumstances. It will not be acceptable not to know anything about your expert subject area or to require continual prompting, rephrasing or repetition of questions, unless the university has put in place reasonable adjustments to support a learning need, for example.

In the vein of supporting your needs on the day, it is quite normal to require hydration, food or a comfort break during your viva. Remember that your examiners are there to help you. If you are uncomfortable, it is important to ask for what you need. Examiners know and appreciate that this is an extremely anxiety-provoking time for students. Indeed, they have been through it themselves, so they understand the feeling more than you know. To support you in the best way, think ahead and have your strategies figured out beforehand, so that you know in advance where the restrooms are and have access to fresh water and food as needed. If you are undertaking the viva using an online platform, the etiquette will be similar; you may request a break with the opportunity to turn off your camera and mute your sound to enable you to drink or take a comfort break.

The duration of the viva varies. My viva took 2.5 hours, but I have heard of some lasting between 4 and 6 hours. The important point here is not to worry about how long it takes. By the day of your viva, you should be prepared with all your home comforts (food and water), so you should have no need to be unduly worried about the length of the viva. In the end, you will be in the room as long as it takes for you to cover the material adequately and discuss it critically. Believe me, you will be grateful for the time you have. The examiners want to give you the opportunity to discuss your work thoroughly, to defend your ideas and your reasoning, so it makes sense that this will take time. This is why preparation is key. If you have all you need in that room and you know you may have breaks as needed, you do not need to worry about how long it will take; you can just be and enjoy it.

For me, my viva was an amazing day of self-actualisation. I was finally becoming who I knew I was. My cup was overflowing; in fact, I found it difficult to stop talking because it was so nice to have a captive audience. This is the thing about a viva: it is your final opportunity to discuss your doctorate from beginning to end, to discuss the barriers and how you navigated them and, most importantly, to celebrate your successes. Having examiners who have specific knowledge that relates to your research is an amazing opportunity. It was energising to be able to really discuss my thesis with people who knew exactly what I was talking about.

Post Viva

Once the viva is finished, the examiners will debate and discuss your performance against the university criteria, with which you will be, by now, extremely familiar. The examiners took approximately 20 minutes to discuss mine, and then they called me into the room again to deliver the verdict. I can honestly say that this was perhaps the most nerve-wracking moment: that moment when you know it's all over and you can do no more.

My lead supervisor kindly agreed to meet with me when I exited the room as the examiners began their discussion. Just knowing that she was there really helped me. I couldn't bring myself to speak and simply paced around the place as my supervisor chatted gently to me. At that point in the process, your supervisors know you almost better than you know yourself; they know what you need, how important it is to you and the sacrifices you have made in order to undertake a doctorate. I knew that the next few moments could change things forever, I had nothing more to give and felt ready for whatever came my way.

After 20 minutes of pacing, the final moment of reckoning arrived. I was invited into the room again. As I took a seat, my heart was beating fast and that feeling of emotion began to well inside me. The examiners were extremely considerate and wasted no time to tell me that I had been successful. The tears that came were a little embarrassing on a professional level, but at this point I was beyond caring.

Doctoral Outcomes

There are several possible outcomes when it comes to a doctorate. Ultimately, you may pass or fail. If you pass, there are then additional categories, which may vary between universities, but usually include the following:

- Pass with no corrections, in which case your work is done and no revisions are required.
- Pass with minor corrections, in which case some minor errors need to be corrected or revised, such as basic typographical errors within the text, graphs or tables.
- Pass with major corrections, in which there are major amendments to be made that could require rewriting a chapter or chapters, for example.

If you have passed, the examiners will then assign you to one of the above categories. They will then take the time to advise you on the university process that follows. For example, I recall being told I passed and then asked to sign papers to confirm that the viva had taken place and that I agreed with the outcome. The examiners and my lead supervisor then signed the same forms. Once those forms were signed, the viva was terminated and the forms were sent to the university.

A Special Day

Although the above process seems quite clinical on paper, the reality is that it was one of the most unforgettable days. I cried many tears of joy that day and even managed to get a photograph of myself with my examiners to commemorate it. Once we left the room, my supervisor announced that she had booked a nice table at a local restaurant to celebrate. I suggest that this is a really nice thing to do if you have the opportunity. As an introvert at heart, I found a nice meal with a small group of interested, experienced researchers the perfect way to celebrate. As we chatted and shared stories, I realised in that moment that the examiners were human beings with families, their own worries and pressures. They were not those people whom I saw standing on a pedestal at conferences or on social media. They were human, and what a relief it was to know this. Remember this as you enter your viva. When it comes to this day, there is more to be celebrated than feared.

Opportunities and Reflections

Since a viva experience is like a rather lengthy interview, unexpected opportunities may result from it. For example, following my viva, I was invited by one of the examiners to visit a small start-up at the University of Oxford to share my research with a community of engineers and also to visit the Netherlands to share my work further and to begin a potential collaboration.

I also felt inspired following the process. After the viva one of the examiners said, 'Remember, one day you will be at this side of the table, examining doctoral students.' This inspired me to think beyond the viva. He also shared a quotation from Isaac Newton: 'Today you stand on the shoulders of giants.' It was such a powerful end to the viva, encouraging me to reflect upon those who paved the way and inspiring me to think about how I could be those shoulders for someone else. As an associate professor, I have never forgotten his words, and to this day I enjoy paying my experiences forward.

Knowing What You Need

In the days that followed my viva, exhilaration inevitably gave way to post-viva exhaustion. It was a type of exhaustion that I had never encountered before. Prior to this, I had experienced over-working and crashing, which I could usually resolve with a weekend of rest, but this was different. Post viva, the exhaustion somehow felt heavier and prolonged. I remember remarking on the way I felt to a close friend of mine who had experienced the same. She told me that it took her nearly 12 months to recover from her doctorate. While I found it difficult to believe that it would take 12 months, I believe that in the end she was correct. After nearly 4 years of a doctoral marathon, I needed to reboot and to look after myself.

Recovery did not mean 'not working'; it simply meant that moving forward I needed to look after myself with a little more compassion. Rather than jumping quickly into the next thing, I undertook a post-doc in a related area. This gave me the opportunity to work part-time hours and therefore remain in research while injecting more time into my family life. It enabled me to enjoy the simple things again, to rest and recover. Grounding myself in what I needed at this time meant that I could get ready for the next stage. It meant that I had time to reflect and to discover what my future research focus would be, the skills that I required and the collaborative team that I needed to work with to make this happen.

It turns out that the greatest learning from my doctorate was not the academic part, but the learning that happens when you are going through the process. It is the survival techniques you learn, knowing yourself and how you work best. It is knowing what you need and doing that, which is the greatest learning of all.

Finding Your Way: Viva Voce – Learning Points

- Viva voce means 'with living voice' and is an oral assessment that is completed by doctoral students following the submission of their theses.
- In advance of the viva, it is vital to consider the criteria and regulations under which you will be examined so that you can prepare well and ensure that you meet the requirements.
- Preparation for the viva voce starts from the beginning of your doctorate, and you will need to take responsibility for this. Embrace opportunities to present and share your research to build the confidence required to communicate and defend your research during your viva.
- Discuss the viva process at your university with trusted post-doctoral peers. Your supervisor may be able to recommend someone to you.
- Plan well. It is important to know what you need and to communicate this with your supervisors to assist planning. Don't forget practicalities such as travel, supplies or the equipment that you may need on the day.
- Think about your setback plan. If you experience issues with travel or have a mental block on the day, how will you deal with this? Always have a plan B.
- If you require reasonable adjustments, do not be discouraged. Simply discuss the adjustments with your supervisors or contact the university disability support services in good time to make a suitable plan.
- Organise a practice viva, if this is possible and works for you.
- During the viva, feel comfortable in asking for what you need (comfort breaks, asking examiners to repeat a question if you cannot hear or understand it, etc.). Enjoy the discussion and sharing your research.
- Bring your thesis with you to support you on the day. Highlighter pens or sticky notes may help you to identify different chapters with ease or may help as a simple aide-mémoire.
- Following the viva, take some time out to recover. If possible, consider flexible working options and avoid taking too much on in this period. Identify what you need and simply do that.
- Take time to consider next steps and celebrate your success!

Finding Your Way: Viva Voce – Action Points

The most important action points that I can act on today/this week/this month are

Finding Your Way Viva Voce – Steps Towards Achieving Action Points

The next steps I can take towards these action points are

CHAPTER 12

Celebrating Success

Colleagues should take of each other, have fun, celebrate success, learn by failure, look for reasons to praise not to criticize, communicate freely and respect each other.
—Richard Branson

I have left the chapter 'Celebration of success' near the end of the first section of this book, largely because this is where people expect to find it – at the end. Throughout the journey, doctoral students expect to celebrate at the end of the process, when all is done, the thesis has been submitted and the viva voce is complete. In this respect I was no different: I imagined how amazing it would all be if I could just get to this point, if I could just get 'there'. However, in my naivety, I failed to recognise that during the doctoral process there is no return or reward for your efforts in the short term. While you may submit your thesis and complete your viva successfully, you never truly get 'there', to that imaginary place where all is well and you feel completely satisfied. As one of my mentors pointed out quite early on in my doctoral experience, once you finish your doctorate and graduate, there will be another academic Everest or challenge ahead of you, not only because you choose it but because this is who you are, curious and equipped to challenge the status quo.

Celebrate Each Win Along the Way

However, there are choices we can make. We can either choose to leave our celebration to the end, when we get 'there', or choose to reframe success by celebrating every win along the way in order to motivate and reward our endeavours as we prepare ourselves for the doctoral long game and future research careers. In my opinion, it is important that the celebration of our success is not left until 'the end' that never arrives. We deserve to celebrate each achievement or win along the way—but how?

To describe what worked best for me in terms of celebrating my successes during the doctoral process, I need to share the donkey and carrot/stick analogy. In this analogy, donkeys are motivated to move forward by one of two methods: The donkey may be motivated to move forward when offered a carrot (positive reinforcement) or when driven by a stick (negative reinforcement). Interestingly, humans appear to behave in a similar manner during the doctoral process. At one end of the spectrum, people are very much 'stick' driven, motivated to move forward in negative ways by underestimating their abilities relative to others, negative self-talk or other negative behaviour. At the other end of the spectrum people appear more 'carrot' led, where the celebration of success becomes a powerful motivational driver.

You may find that you operate in either of these two zones or somewhere on the carrot/stick continuum during your doctoral journey. For example, in the first phase of my doctorate, I fell very much into the stick-driven mentality. This approach was familiar to me, and reflecting on this further, I have come to understand that this was the way in which I, rightly or wrongly, interpreted phrases from my upbringing such as 'get on with it', 'do your best', or, as a famous sportswear company encourages us, 'just do it'. By engaging solidly in what I now recognise as sometimes punishing and relentless doctoral action, I believed I could not fail. After all, this approach worked during my undergraduate and master's level education, so why wouldn't it work now? However, while this approach worked for a time, I realised that it was unsustainable on this long haul. It was clear that while during my MSc I could work with little reward in the short term, if I were to go the distance and succeed on my doctoral path, there was only one approach that would work. The carrot would be the only way forward: rewarding and celebrating each success or mini-win along the way.

However, the wins I am talking about are not the successes that are traditionally celebrated. They are the small steps, such as the day you submit a paper, recruit your first patient after months of ethics applications or get to the end of a difficult week. By reframing success in this way, everything becomes that little bit brighter and lighter as you begin to appreciate yourself and give yourself credit for small achievements and take small steps towards doctoral completion.

When I began to reframe success through the celebration of mini-wins, my repertoire of celebratory skills was quite limited, as I was not used to congratulating myself in this way. At first it seemed so self-indulgent. However, as time advanced, I realised that I needed to learn these skills in order to continue on this path. I began by observing what others did. I would notice post-doctoral researchers in my laboratory going out for drinks or coffee to celebrate the end of their working week. Through discussion with peers, I learned that there were an infinite number of ways one could celebrate these mini-wins: a quiet bath, a nice walk, some rest. As they shared their ways, it became clear that I needed to find mine. I needed to create a celebratory repertoire that worked for me.

My celebratory repertoire was quite honestly nonexistent at the beginning of my doctorate, simply because this was not something that I was accustomed to doing. Therefore, I gave myself permission to try it all and to enjoy the process of discovery. Looking for 'the best' way of doing this and not knowing how, I read. However, as I trawled the web and wandered through some of the most beautiful bookshops in London, I found it almost impossible to find any books that met the brief within the healthcare research realm. With time I realised that the only way I was going to learn how to do this was if I reached beyond the traditional research texts and stepped out into the unknown by reading and learning from those who managed to persist and complete their respective Everests despite the challenges they encountered.

It was of interest to me that almost no motivational texts appeared where they needed to be, in a section for healthcare professionals in research, but instead they were to be found in the business, sport and psychology sections of my favourite bookshops. Although I found this to some extent surprising, I recognised that sometimes it is necessary to read outside of your own scope of practice, particularly when you are attempting to do new things and enter uncharted personal and professional territories.

Most of the inspirational books that I read were designed for people from business backgrounds. Yet when I picked them apart, I realised that these findings could have implications for healthcare professionals in research. The messages were clear and the skills transferrable. Therefore, I used these ideas as a starting block from which to create my own repertoire. I respected the fact that not all suggestions would work for me, but this was OK, because I was learning and I simply needed to start somewhere.

As I read, I soon established that rewards did not simply need to be something that happened after an event. Boring tasks could be accompanied by a concurrent reward, such as listening to music or working from home. I learned that I could choose particular achievements to add up to a very special reward, such as a day trip or a day off. I could even select a celebratory reward that encouraged productivity, such as meeting with my supervisory team in a coffee shop rather than a traditional location.

On this journey, I have found that rewards are best when they are well considered. By identifying what you need to achieve or reflecting upon what you have achieved, it will be possible to focus the reward for maximum benefit. For example, reflecting upon the past month, you may have identified that you have worked hard and are exhausted as a result. Therefore, to reward your efforts, you may choose to rejuvenate by pencilling in some well needed rest to celebrate.

While sometimes just being able to tick things off a list is motivation enough, towards the end of your doctorate, and beyond, having something concrete to look forward to is helpful. Lists, diaries or charts can act as a helpful visual reminder of your progress and can be used to plan your rewards. Rather as with holidays, if you have nothing in the diary, it can feel that there is nothing positive on the horizon. Therefore, I encourage you to celebrate every moment, and to plan your rewards by identifying opportunities for celebration. Although not an exhaustive list, here are a few reasons to celebrate:

- Getting through a challenging supervision meeting
- Abstract or publication acceptance
- Presenting at a conference
- Writing or submitting a paper
- Finishing data collection
- Completing a section of or submitting your thesis
- The first or final time that you do anything on your doctoral journey

Celebrating Success on Difficult Days

To illustrate how important celebrating your successes is, I find it interesting to think back upon the final year of my doctorate. Initially, as you enter into the heavier writing stage of your final doctoral year, it is exciting. You begin to organise your chapters in the way you have been visualising them for the longest time. As your thesis skeleton develops, it feels satisfying to organise your pre-published papers and table of contents. However, the time eventually comes when you can no longer avoid pulling together the discussion and overarching conclusions of your work. For myself, when the inevitable challenge of argument development, critical analysis and communicating my unique contribution to global research in the field came, I cannot deny feeling overwhelmed. I felt the weight of producing a piece of meaningful and impactful work for funders, stakeholders and the university and ultimately a piece of writing that I could be proud of.

As the feeling of being overwhelmed grows and you are writing every day, it is easy for negative self-talk to invade. At this point you may feel tired and tempted to drive yourself forwards using scalding words of negative self-talk or to procrastinate with a Netflix series. Don't get me wrong: brainless activities have their place. However, in general, days like this are not good for the soul, and often small and gentle action in the right direction of travel is required. This is why scheduling writing sprints and celebrating mini-writing successes can really help during this phase.

Each morning I found it useful to plan my goals for the day. I usually set three achievable goals and simultaneously planned the celebration of each. On good days, when I finished writing a chapter, for example, I would celebrate this success by finishing a little early on that day and cooking with my family. On a difficult day, when the words just did not come so easily, I needed to remind myself that there would be days like this and that tomorrow was another day. On these days I found it useful to rejuvenate with a nice bath, a walk in a nearby forest or a virtual yoga class. If you are having a similar experience, you may find that simply prescribing yourself the carrots you need will help you to find the motivation to cross that finish line.

Graduation Day

During my doctorate, I regularly walked to my university past the Royal Albert Hall in London, where all of the doctoral graduations took place. Walking by this ancient, rotund building, miles high and emblazoned with gold figures, I wondered if I would ever be invited through those regal gates to celebrate my graduation. However, once you are on the doctoral path, the train has very much left the station and inevitably you will begin to visualise graduation day; believing that graduation is no longer just a possibility, it is becoming more of a certainty for you.

However, the day of my graduation was not quite as I had visualised in my mind. On the morning of my graduation I recall sitting with my young boys as I had my breakfast. I could hear the rain hitting the velux windows in our London flat, a sound I usually loved, but not on that day. My mum's diagnosis of late-stage Parkinson's imposed its own challenges, but thanks to my university, I was able to invite my mum and family to celebrate with me virtually. Meanwhile, my dad had bought tickets to fly over to London to celebrate with my husband and me in person.

I pre-ordered my cap and gown from my University as advised, and when they arrived on my doorstep, I knew that my life would never be the same again. I recall the weight of the gown and the pride with which I wore it on that day of celebration. Somehow it did not matter who was there or not there or whether the rain poured or it did not. On this day, the memories of the journey, those who paved the way, family members who never had this opportunity, flooded my head. As I took my place in the Royal Albert hall, I did not move; I simply soaked it all in and chose to celebrate my success.

As each doctoral student filed towards the stage to receive their certificate, I noted that everyone shook hands with the president of the university and said 'Thank you'. However, somehow these words did not seem right for me. As I approached the stage, my heart thumping, I realised that I could not say these words because they were not enough to describe how much this experience had shaped me and changed my family history and would enable me to do the work I was born to do. In that moment, as I shook the president's hand, I leant forward and whispered, 'This will change my life,' and it really did.

Celebrating Success

Sharing success is not easy for everyone. As we learn to share in research, it may feel awkward. Indeed, this is the way I felt, as in my culture, sharing success is often interpreted as a boastful exercise. Indeed, I am quite sure we can all think of times when we have worked within a culture where sharing success just simply is not on the agenda. It almost seems that there is 'no time' for success. In my experience of working within such cultures, the enthusiasm to work at the very best level wanes when success cannot be celebrated. When results or outcomes remain uncelebrated, then it simply doesn't matter whether you do a good job or not. In this type of culture, the entire team is affected, morale depletes, and quite honestly, it affects people's staying power.

However, as you progress through your research career, you realise that it is important to share success, not in order to boast, but to encourage, support and celebrate upcoming researchers, colleagues and your team. In fact, increasingly, universities and funders are supporting researchers sharing success stories in order to foster collaboration and networking, to share knowledge and to engage with stakeholders and inspire people. If you think about it, how many times have you heard of success within your own research or clinical setting and been inspired by it, thinking that perhaps this could be your story too? If we share our stories of research success, perhaps we break down the barriers for our respective communities, making research somehow more accessible and inclusive.

In my career there have been many amazing people who, by sharing their successes, have shown me what could be possible if I dared to dream it. Somehow, I always knew I was different and that my career was unlike that of many of my colleagues. If I dared to dream it and was honest with myself, I wanted to be a professor. However, I could not say the words or express it, feeling that it might somehow be misconstrued as boastful or 'Who does she think she is?' During these times, as I sat quietly with these feelings of knowing where I wanted to go and not quite knowing how to get there, I listened for the voices that resonated with me. I listened to the way in which they shared their successes and lifted others. From these experiences, I could appreciate how sharing generously in this way had knock-on effects on individuals and entire teams, boosting confidence, creating energy and encouraging a culture where success is to be celebrated and not denied.

Share Your Success Your Way

Although it is important to share success to inspire and support the next generation, I have learned that it is also important to share in your own way. By that I mean to share in a way that you feel comfortable with. For myself, I have found that I am only happy to share my successes when it feels comfortable to do so and in line with my values. Doing it your way means that you express yourself authentically and using a medium that you feel most comfortable with, be it through social media, written publications or face-to-face interactions.

Knowing what to share is important. For myself, I like to share publications, funding successes and failures and opportunities for students to learn and grow and choose to celebrate the successes of my research colleagues, collaborators, stakeholders, students and patients. For me, this aligns with my values. Anything that does not support others, cannot be shared or does not inspire is not for me.

As we learn to share our success, we sometimes share naively and without purpose, or overshoot by sharing too much. It is true that people do not always appreciate it when people share success after success after success, while they are experiencing the inevitable failures that life brings. However, the same is true if we elect to drone on about our failures, which may be interpreted as negative rants and make for depressing reading. For these reasons, whether we are sharing our successes or failures, we need to think about our purpose. Why do you wish to share a particular success or failure? What difference will this make to your community?

Dealing With Negativity

As you celebrate and share your successes, you may experience some negativity. Although I have generally not experienced this on social media, since I choose to engage with professional research communities, it is possible that you may encounter jealousy or unkind comments. In these rare instances, I think it is a good rule of thumb to resist engaging with such individuals on social media. They don't deserve your time and attention, so ignore the negativity, disengage and block those that do not serve you or your community in the best way.

Sometimes negativity can occur when you least expect it. In the final phase of my doctorate I was invited to share my research-capacity-building experiences at a professional event. At the time I had created a research platform to support the next generation of healthcare professionals in research. I was excited to share my preliminary work experiences and to celebrate the success of the multidisciplinary team who helped me to develop it. As it was a new style of conference with which I was unfamiliar and the audience was new, I was a little nervous. However, as I took the courage to present my work, a lady dressed in a suit stared at my presentation and without introducing herself said, 'Well, I could do this; in fact, I think I could do this better.' She promptly took pictures of my presentation, including the methods, results and references, and walked off. Deflated and dumbfounded, I stood there thinking: if this is the community into which I am walking, I am not sure that this is for me. However, like waves rushing to shore, her negativity was soon washed away by new, fresh comments from an audience of enthusiastic and encouraging minds. In this instance, I chose to bathe in positive waters, ignoring the negative ripples created by this unwelcome guest.

Although as a researcher you will certainly encounter challenge, and will be required to defend your ideas, you should be able to share your work in a safe space where people respect your ambition and your success and offer constructive comments. However, in reality, it does not always work like this. So when you encounter challenges, I encourage you to remember why you are sharing your research, your values and your intentions as you share. Waves of negativity will soon pass and good will prevail if you let it.

Sharing Failures

Sharing failures is not easy. I think this is largely because we fear the way in which people may interpret our failures. Certainly, as I was growing up, failure was not an option at school. The prize was awarded for success, never recognising the journey of successive failures that it took to get there. By not sharing our failures, it sometimes feels to me as if we are short-changing the next generation. We are almost setting them up with the idea that success is the only way, that success is achievable with what appears to be minimum effort and that failure does not feature on the pathway towards success.

Last week I found it interesting to observe the experience of failure from the perspective of my 11-year-old son. At my son's school, each week a child is selected to bring home the 'Science bag' and to design an experiment. Although it is a parent's dread to have a last-minute piece of extra homework to deal with, it turned out to be a great learning experience. As we peered into the bag, we realised that there was no end to the type of experiments that he could choose to do. In the end, he selected two Petri dishes and decided to examine the growth of bacteria using swabs taken from his Dad's phone and, yes, our toilet.

From the outset, his hypothesis was that yes, Dad's phone would be more bacterially infested than our toilet. To undertake the experiment, we needed agar jelly, which we bought from the chemist. Not reading the contents of the packet, I filled each Petri dish with agar, as instructed. Once the agar had solidified, my son then spread the bacteria-laden swabs across the agar. We carefully considered the conditions to encourage maximum growth and watched and waited as my son tabulated the progress. However, the table did not make for happy reading, as from day 1 to 4 the table read 'no growth'. By day 7, my son was upset understanding, that the experiment had officially failed and that he had nothing to share other than one photo of an empty Petri dish and one table that noted 'no growth'. As I would later establish, I sadly failed to notice that the agar jelly was devoid of nutrients, so our bacteria had no hope of growing. However, despite this epic Mum fail, we began to discuss the importance of experimental failure and why sometimes failure tells us more about where we need to focus our efforts in order to succeed next time.

As every experienced researcher appreciates, failure is a very necessary part of the journey towards success. Not only does failure direct our next steps, but it is through experiencing failure that we begin to appreciate our successes more completely. For myself, I often find it helpful to share my failures alongside my successes. In this way, people understand that success is possible in the wake of failure. However, sharing it my way means that I only share my personal failures when I feel safe and comfortable to do so. This usually occurs when I present in person at invited talks or conferences, wheren I can see and interact personally with people, where the cost of sharing and being vulnerable will have the most impact and inspire others.

As a mentor and supervisor, I also like to share honestly and openly with my students so that they have a realistic picture of the road ahead. Although, being an introvert, it is not always easy for me to share failures in this way, I do so because the cost of not doing it is greater for my community in the long term. As healthcare professionals in research who have the privilege of undertaking a doctorate, I believe we should embrace and celebrate our successes and failures and feel comfortable in celebrating this messiness as part of our authentic research journey.

Finding Your Way: Celebrating Success – Learning Points

- Celebrate each and every win in your way.
- Reward small achievements or mini-wins by establishing a personal repertoire.
- Thoughtfully consider the reward that will work best for you in a given scenario. Will a concurrent reward, such as playing music as you organise your inbox, work best, or will the reward of rest help more after a busy doctoral day?
- Identify opportunities for small celebrations, such as finishing data collection or writing up a thesis chapter for review.
- Once you have identified opportunities for celebration, plan your rewards in advance. In this way, you can look forward to it and enjoy the buildup.
- On a difficult doctoral day, try setting three achievable goals and plan a celebratory reward following the completion of each. This will help to motivate you.
- Share your success your way. Share only when it feels comfortable and safe to do so. Ensure that what you share aligns with your values. Avoid engaging with negativity.
- When sharing your successes or failures, consider your intention and purpose for sharing. How will it serve your research community?
- Through sharing the inevitable successes and failures in your way, you share the authentic and necessary journey towards doctoral success that will inspire future generations.

Finding Your Way: Celebrating Success – Action Points

The most important action points that I can act on today/this week/this month are

Finding Your Way: Celebrating Success – Steps Towards Achieving Action Points

The next steps I can take towards these action points are

CHAPTER 13

Paying It Forward

Leveraging your privilege and paying it forward encourages cross-cultural and cross-experiential empathy, providing authentic opportunities to see beyond the professional persona and connect with people on a more personal level. By doing so, we can destigmatise privilege and unlock its potential instead.
—Jacqueline Ferguson

When the dust has settled and you have received your doctorate, it is inevitable to think what's next. However, if we stand still and reflect on the journey, we soon realise how privileged we are. The privilege to learn, to write, to engage and collaborate in research should not be underestimated. Now as we move forward, we are in a different position from where we began, and it is important to acknowledge this.

In the first year of my doctorate, I attended a presentation by a well-known professor from University of Cambridge. The presentation represented a reflection on his research journey, experiences and subsequent success. As the professor stood behind the podium, he eloquently shared the truth of his success in research, which he attributed to three elements: a set of binary decisions, curiosity and a lot of luck.

The binary decisions that he described related to that moment where you have 'yes' or 'no' decisions to make: to accept a job offer or not, to do a doctorate or not. At the time he was a father of young children; therefore, he decided that each binary decision would be made on the basis of whether or not it worked for his family. While this made sure that each decision was both acceptable and sustainable for his family, success would also be determined by his undeniable and relentless curiosity.

Although it seemed reasonable that decision-making and curiosity should underpin a successful research career, it was a leap for me to accept that luck was responsible for the majority of his success. We may be curious and make good decisions, but at the end of the day, is it all down to luck? However, as I progress in my career, I realise that there were wisdom and honesty in his words. It is luck indeed that affords us our unique privilege as doctoral students. It is our privilege that we have gotten to this point, that we have received the necessary support, mentorship, education and financial backing to make this opportunity possible. Now as graduates and custodians of this doctoral privilege it is important that we share this and pay our experiences forward.

Everyone Needs a Champion

In my career so far, I have observed the destruction that unhappiness brings, how resentment related to difficult doctoral experiences can pass from generation to generation as researchers teach as they have been taught. Often researchers behave in this way because they have suffered extreme neglect as part of their personal doctoral process. Perhaps they have experienced absentee professors or a personal lack of support or empathy and were expected to fend for themselves during their doctorates. In this old system of doctoral supervision, graduates learned that this neglect and fending for oneself were a rite of passage. In this way, researchers could continue simply to teach as they had been taught, using the school of hard knocks as their foundation. However, it does not have to be this way. As you now move towards becoming a supervisor in your own right, it will be your choice as to which type of supervisor you become.

In my life, I choose differently. I choose optimism and to let go of experiences that have not served me or others well. At different times and in different universities, I can say that I have experienced an entire spectrum of supervision and mentorship: some amazing, some tear-initiating. Fortunately, when you graduate, you get to choose the research leader that you would like to become. When you do, it is important to take the time to consider your values, what type of leader you will be and who you will celebrate and support moving forward. You will do so in the knowledge that your past experiences of what 'a researcher' is like do not need to define your future leadership style. Through detailed consideration of your values as a future research leader, you can transform the experiences of others and choose to lead differently.

In my opinion, effective research leadership requires personal reflection, authenticity, generosity and compassion. In the case of my doctorate, my lead supervisor was quite special. She supported my growth and shared networking opportunities and contacts with me. It always seemed that if she did not know how, she knew someone who could help me. She gave me space to experiment as an adult learner and yet was always there to chat when times were tough. Given this positive experience, I learned a lot about the future research leader I could become.

Later I came to learn from a research friend and professor that all doctoral students need that person in their corner: someone to champion and support their work as they grow. He always said, 'everyone needs a fairy godmother or godfather in research,' and my supervisor epitomised this. To this day I cannot thank her enough for supporting the earliest stages of my career and being my champion. As we grow old together and meet for walks and coffees, I always share that I simply would not be where I am without her.

Values

Growing up, I was taught to believe that leaders needed to be hard, tough and extroverted, but now I am learning that leaders can be softer, quieter and more empathic. In fact, as a healthcare professional in research, it is important to remember that as a leader it is important to be authentically yourself. I only truly recognised this when I undertook a course in leadership sponsored by my professional society. During this course, I was encouraged to understand who I was as a leader and team player. I filled out the obligatory questionnaire to have it confirmed that yes, I am a natural leader, team player and at the heart of it all, an introvert. Through this process I learned that being an introvert meant that I was not shy but rather I gain my energy from quiet spaces, unlike extroverts who gain their energy from noisy and crowded environments. I subsequently read a lot of Susan Cain's work on introversion (see Resources) and gained confidence that I could absolutely lead just as I am. I did not need to be loud or to shout, or to lead as I was led; I had the potential to be a leader in research just as I was.

During the leadership course I also learned the importance of establishing my values. Opportunities to reflect inspired me to think about who I was and what was most important to me as a research leader. As I sat with my notebook and pen, the words flowed and my values became clear and could be summarised in three simple words: support, share and inspire. Slowly I began to use these three words to describe what I did and what I wished for future generations of healthcare leaders in research. These values became so central to my work that when I designed and developed a national support community for healthcare professionals in research in the United Kingdom, I threaded these values throughout the content and used them to support decision-making. In fact, to this day, these values infuse everything I do.

Celebrating and Supporting the Next Generation in Clinical Research

As a doctoral graduate, you will begin to lead new projects and become part of collaborative work. However, the largely unspoken responsibility of doctoral graduates is, I believe, to celebrate and support the next generation. It is critical to the development of future clinical academic careers that we pay our privilege forward so that nobody 'goes it alone'; rather, we become a diverse community of researchers working together to do important work for the benefit of our patients and the societies in which we live.

Practically there are many ways in which you could celebrate and support the next generation, but again, this is not always acknowledged within the literature. It seems that most books like to focus on getting you through the doctorate but don't consider what you might like to do when you get there. However, I am keen that we shouldn't waste our most valuable resource, our success stories and our experiences.

Boundaries

When you begin to celebrate and support others, expect to either overshoot and share/support too much or undershoot and share/support too little. This is all part of the process as you find your way. Remember that you are a precious resource that cannot fire on empty, so while you feel encouraged to share and inspire, there should be some defined boundaries in your plan as you prepare to pay your privilege forward. This may require defining the number of hours that you are willing to devote to supporting external committees or certain days when you agree to share information with new researchers on social media. Whatever way you choose to share, make sure it is meaningful, supportive and above all sustainable.

Becoming a Supervisor or Mentor

When you finish your doctorate, one of the first ways in which you may choose to share, support and inspire is by becoming a doctoral supervisor or mentor. There are certain building blocks that need to be in place before you start. First, universities usually provide courses for doctoral supervisors so that they are equipped with the resources and education required to ensure the best student experience and outcome. When you begin, you may find it useful to become a co-supervisor for a doctoral student and then advance to be a lead supervisor when you feel more confident and proficient. It is usual for each doctoral student to be supervised by more than one supervisor, and this can really help when you begin. Of course, this is just one example of how you may choose to pay our privilege forward, but there are many ways. To inspire you, here are a few ideas:

- Become a research mentor or champion.
- Join a committee that supports grass roots research activity. This could include funding bodies, charitable trusts or councils.
- Network with doctoral students and early career researchers at conferences.
- Reach out directly to people from underrepresented groups in research. Could they become part of your research community, committee or group?
- Supervise undergraduate, masters, pre-doctoral or doctoral research students.
- Offer student research projects. Involving students in your research is one way to improve student confidence and self-belief.
- Share your experiences with doctoral students at meetings, conferences and invited talks. By sharing honestly and with integrity, you will be relatable and pave the way for others to do the same.

- Write and disseminate your research experiences through simple tips, publications and blogs.
- Support students on social media by liking or retweeting or following their content.
- Co-author publications with research students.
- Register for funding committees so that you become aware of the funding landscape and can support students with future funding applications.
- Share job opportunities using adverts that are encouraging and inclusive.
- Set up a local research community to support research activity or early career researchers if one does not already exist.

Pay It Forward

As my viva voce determined, I was not at the viva because of my sole determination and hard work; I was there because of the many clinical researchers who had paved the way, those who lifted me, championed my research and supported me. I was there because of my privilege.

Now that you have completed your doctorate, I invite you to consider who you will lift and how you will pay your privilege forward. I respect that sometimes this is not easy. This is particularly the case if your doctoral supervision has not been as you would have liked or if you needed to forge your way ahead alone without mentorship or support because there was no guiding light. However, we are in a position to change the future narrative and research culture. Who could you lift, walk alongside and support today?

Finding Your Way: Paying It Forward – Learning Points

- As a doctoral graduate, it is important to recognise your privilege and to think about ways in which you could pay your experiences forward for the benefit of your profession and the patients you serve.
- As a doctoral graduate, it is important to reflect on the support and inspiration you needed to get you through your studies before beginning to pay your experiences forward.
- To guide you, reflect on both the positive and negative doctoral experiences you have had. This will help you to define the future research leader that you would like to become.
- Lead authentically, generously and with compassion. Not everyone needs to lead in the same way. Consider what your values are and how you like to lead and gain feedback from colleagues to inform your approach.
- As a doctoral graduate, it will be your responsibility to celebrate and support the next generation. Don't waste your most valuable resource: your success stories and experiences. Share them.
- Share and support in your way. Define boundaries to ensure that you can sensibly commit to the support you are offering. Share in ways that are meaningful to you and your profession, making sure they are sustainable in the long term.
- There are many ways in which you can pay your privilege forward, including supervision, mentorship, committee membership and allyship.
- When there is no guiding light, become your own and reach out. If the support is not there, reach out through your professional networks and social media.
- Who could you lift, walk alongside and support today?

Finding Your Way: Paying It Forward – Action Points

The most important action points that I can act on today/this week/this month are

Finding Your Way: Paying It Forward – Steps Towards Achieving Action Points

The next steps I can take towards these action points are

Interviews With Experienced Healthcare Professionals Involved in Research

The only source of knowledge is experience.

—ALBERT EINSTEIN

CHAPTER 14

Overview of Interviews With Experienced Healthcare Professionals in Research

In this section, I interview an inspiring group of healthcare professionals about their personal doctoral experiences. The aim of this section is to add breadth and depth to the personal reflections I shared in Section One.

Each chapter in Section Two reflects the chapters explored in the previous section, so that you can read my experiences and then explore another perspective. As you read, you will note the similarities, the threads of experience that we share and the hurdles that we encounter on the way. Although we come from different healthcare professions and may have different doctoral experiences, in the end the journey is very much the same.

The interviewees represent a diverse set of professional backgrounds and career stages and have shared generously and honestly to support your doctoral journey. I hope that you enjoy reading about their doctoral experiences and top tips as much as I did.

CHAPTER 15

Undertaking a Professional Doctorate

Interview with Professor Jane Simmonds (Paediatric Physiotherapy)

1. In your experience, what is a typical doctoral journey like?

The professional doctorate structure varies from subject to subject and institution to institution. They are usually undertaken over a 5–6-year period while also working. Common to all professional doctorates is the completion of an original piece of research and, in my case, the additional creation of a professional product (an educational training video for physical education teacher). The research is presented as a thesis and is examined by experts in the specialist field. Usually, the research project relates to real-life issues concerned with professional practice and often carried out within the student's own organisation. Professional doctorate candidates often use their current knowledge and abilities to develop interests and become change-makers within their communities of practice and within their professional areas.

2. How did your journey differ from the typical journey?

Unlike a PhD programme, my professional doctorate started with writing a critical evaluation of my professional practice. The review was a structured piece of work which included an analysis of research experience, clinical practice and education activities. This evaluation allowed me to develop the major themes of my doctoral studies and research. The next step in the process involved completing taught modules in research methods, leadership and change management which then led to the development of my major research projects. The taught modules were assessed via course work essays and the final thesis comprised of my research with a critical commentary of the potential impact of my projects on clinical and education practice and my plans for implementing change.

3. What was the advantage of undertaking a professional doctorate for you?

As a pragmatist, the professional doctorate route was right for me because it enabled me to draw together my passion for education and clinical practice while facilitating research and leadership knowledge and skills. The work-based nature of the doctorate allowed me to continue to work full time and to contribute and lead in my workplace.

4. In your opinion, what should people consider before undertaking a doctorate?

I think the timing of a doctorate is very personal. It is very important to appreciate the mental, emotional and time commitment before starting out. Resilience, perseverance and support are needed for a successful completion. For some people, an early research career is perfect, and for others it is important to have professional experience prior to starting. Undertaking a professional doctorate such as mine requires several years of professional work in order to establish myself as an educator and clinical specialist while also understanding the complexities of professional organisations.

5. How did you select your doctoral research theme and overarching research question?

Through the process of the initial critical reflection on my professional practice, it became very clear to me that my interests were in the 'hidden disorders' of osteoporosis and hypermobility syndromes. My first doctoral research study was opportunistic and explored the impact of stair climbing on bone health and behaviour change in pre- and post-menopausal women. The project was undertaken in the institution where I worked, taking advantage of one of the elevator's being refurbished. My primary supervisor quite simply wondered: What happens to bone turnover when women who are usually sedentary start to climb stairs on a regular basis? The second project related to my first degree in physical education and my experience of working with children with symptomatic hypermobility. I had identified a need through my clinical work for physical education teacher to be aware of how joint hypermobility might impact on skill development, sports performance and injury in children. I therefore asked the question: How will a hypermobility training programme impact the knowledge and practice of PE teachers in a secondary school?

6. What support was available to you in the pre-doctoral and doctoral phases?

Prior to the doctorate, I talked to senior clinical and academic colleagues, my partner and engaged in academic career development seminars at the university where I worked. This helped me to decide on the type of doctorate I wanted to do. I was very fortunate to obtain financial support and study time support from the universities where I worked while undertaking the doctorate. Additionally, I obtained small financial research and project grants from a local education authority and the Musculoskeletal Association of Chartered Physiotherapists to support the research projects and assist with dissemination.

7. In your experience, how has this changed with time?

Since completing my doctorate 13 years ago, there is much more support for healthcare professionals to help steer an academic path and create networks. The NIHR fellowship programmes have enabled talented research-minded professionals to access research careers. The Council for Allied Health Professions Research has also provided excellent support for research professional development. Moreover, social media platforms such as Twitter facilitate excellent communications about research and professional support opportunities.

8. How did you feel after submitting your thesis and completing your viva?

There was a huge sense of relief and sense of validation. I had doubts prior to submitting my thesis as to whether I had done enough and whether the work was novel enough. I didn't know anyone else who had done a professional doctorate in my field, and therefore I had no benchmark. Due to the nature of my doctorate, there was more work to do, as I needed to publish my physical education training video training programme and push forward and lead in the education and research of physiotherapists and health professionals in hypermobility-related conditions and osteoporosis.

9. How did undertaking a doctorate influence your practice and career trajectory?

Completing my doctorate had a profound influence of on all spheres of my professional life. The impact has been far greater than I ever expected. In all three areas of my professional life - clinical practice, education and research – I have been able to continue to advance and grow due to the knowledge, skills and confidence developed through the doctoral process. Towards the end of my doctorate, I became a programme leader of an MSc Programme and was promoted to Professional Lead for Physiotherapy at the University of Hertfordshire, and I was part of the leadership team which created the London Hypermobility Unit. Due to the nature of my major project which involved adolescents, I shifted my professional practice to focus more on child health. This led to an opportunity to move to University College London, Great Ormond Street Institute of Child Health where I have flourished and thoroughly enjoyed an amazing career teaching students who are passionate about child health, researching and working with outstanding individuals.

10. What are your top three tips for undertaking doctoral research?

1. Undertake a deep and honest analysis of your strengths, interests and ambitions and reflect upon your limitations. This will help you to choose the type of doctorate you want to undertake and help you to focus on the themes and questions.

2. Find a host institution and supervisory team which align to your values. Undertaking a doctorate and working with your team is a big commitment and is like finding a life partner. Values underpin the stability and success of the partnership.

3. Be open to change and examine your motives. The doctoral journey is an opportunity for deep reflection, learning and self-development. If you are open to this wonderful opportunity, anything will be possible!

Jane Simmonds is Professor of Physiotherapy and Health Education at University College London. Originally from Perth, Western Australia, Professor Simmonds completed undergraduate and postgraduate education at the University of Western Australia and Curtin University prior to coming to London where she has lived and worked since 1992. She worked in the National Health Services, occupational health, private practice, elite sport and higher education before completing a Professional Doctorate in Health Studies at Middlesex University where she focussed on advancing professional practice in hidden diseases. Professor Simmonds combines her academic role at UCL Great Ormond Street Institute of Child Health, where she is Co-Director of Education and Programme Lead for the MSc Paediatric Physiotherapy with clinical work as the clinical lead at the Central Health Physiotherapy, London Hypermobility Unit. She is Chair of the Ehlers Danlos Society International Consortium Allied Health working group, a member of the Ehlers Danlos Society Medical and Scientific Board and medical advisor to EDS Support UK, HMSA and PoTS UK.

Professor Simmonds supervises and examines PhD students and has successfully supervised over 100 MSc student projects. She has authored more than 100 research and clinical education publications including peer-reviewed journal articles, book chapters, and patient and clinical guides. Furthermore, she has delivered over 150 national and international invited lectures and keynote presentations, webinars and courses. Professor Simmonds is a Senior Fellow of the Health Education Academy and is the recipient of multiple research and education grants and several education excellence awards. Current collaborative research includes the development of a ballet-specific functional screening tool, creation of a multi-systemic outcome measure for hypermobility-related problems, development of a decision-making tool for children with symptomatic hypermobility, exercise intervention for people with postural orthostatic tachycardia syndrome (PoTS) and investigating upper cervical instability in people with Hypermobility Spectrum Dorsers and Hypermobile Ehlers Danlos Syndrome.

CHAPTER 16

Applying for Doctoral Funding and Learning From Experience

Interview with Dr Margaret Coffey (Speech and Language Therapy)

1. **Although doctorates can be self-funded, in many cases people need funding to complete a doctorate. How did you gain funding for your doctorate?**
I received funding from the NIHR Clinical Doctoral Fellowship programme in 2010. This funding stream was developed to support registered health and care practitioners to participate in research.

2. **Did you have mentors to support you in the process?**
Yes, my mentors were critical in supporting me to undertake a PhD and embark on a clinical academic career pathway. When I was thinking about a PhD, I was fortunate to work at an NHS trust which had a dedicated therapies research facilitator, a dietician with both a PhD and an established research career. This person encouraged me to develop my research proposal, apply for funding and helped to prepare me for a NIHR interview.

3. **How did you prepare for making the funding application?**
I really focussed on this. I took opportunities to participate in any research opportunities around me. This included relatively straightforward tasks such as potential participants to review consent forms or undertaking some basic data collection. I drew on this experience for my application to illustrate that I had a basic understanding of what is involved in research. I took some courses on literature searching and critical appraisal to demonstrate a commitment to research skills development.

   I reviewed the evidence base and spoke with my patient population to help identify a research question that was novel but also clinically relevant with potential to improve function. I asked more experienced researchers to review my application to help refine my research proposal. I sought advice to help me write the personal statement section of the application so that I came across as someone who could deliver a PhD and had the potential to become a future clinical academic leader.

4. **As healthcare professionals in research, which transferrable skills do we have to support us with this?**
We have many skills which are transferrable to research which are not always recognised. We are especially good at listening to the perspectives of our patients, which can help with co-design of research proposals. This skill also supports patient and public involvement activities, an essential component of contemporary research.

5. **How much time does it take to prepare an average funding application?**
In my opinion, a PhD funding application takes around 12 months to prepare. I think it is better to take time to submit a really well-prepared application rather than submitting an application that is not quite ready.

6. In your experience, what are the key challenges that people experience?

In pursuing a clinical academic career, the key challenges are often around a lack of understanding of the benefits of research. It's essential to find a way to engage with your clinical/service manager and communicate the benefits of research and outline how these align with NHS strategy at a national level. It's also important to be aware that backfill and recruitment can be a challenge when a team member is awarded funded time for research.

7. There are a range of funding pathways available. What do people need to consider before selecting which funding pathway to take?

Carefully read guidance notes from funding agencies to ensure your project falls within remit. Check whether your research aligns with any themed funding calls. Consider which funding options are best for your project and seek advice from research mentors about this. Think about the scale of your project and how much it is likely to cost. Some funding agencies have limits on how much they will fund for an individual project. It is usually a good idea to consider different funding agencies including professional organisations, and charities in addition to the National Institute of Health Research (NIHR) and the Medical Research Council (MRC).

8. What happens if you apply for funding and fail? Is it possible to resubmit?

A critical part of being a clinical academic means sometimes not being successful when you apply for funding. Most funders will provide useful feedback when a submission has not been successful. If you are unsuccessful with a funding application, take some time out to reflect, consider feedback and look at your options. It is often possible to resubmit an application. However, some funding institutions, such as the NIHR, may place a limit on the number of reapplications you can submit, so check the guidance notes for your funding agency.

9. Have you ever failed to obtain funding? If so, what did you do next?

I have been both successful and unsuccessful in obtaining research funding. When I was unsuccessful, I took time to consider any feedback provided, accessed expert advice and resolved not to become discouraged by failure. Essentially, I picked myself up, dusted myself off and prepared a new application!

10. What are your top three funding tips?

It is difficult to narrow down tips to just three, but here goes!

1. Carefully read and follow any guidance notes provided by the funding agency.
2. Take time to cost the study (including relevant training) comprehensively and accurately. Get help with this as needed.
3. Choose supervisors or research mentors who have the right expertise for your study and are committed to supporting your career as a clinical academic.

Dr Margaret Coffey is a speech and language therapist with extensive experience in the evaluation and treatment of dysphagia arising from multiple aetiologies. She is especially interested in the rehabilitation of communication and swallowing after laryngectomy and other head and neck cancers, the use of fibreoptic endoscopic evaluation of swallowing (FEES) in multidisciplinary clinical practice and evidence-based management of dysphagia. Dr Coffey has developed her clinical skills working in recognised centres of excellence in both the UK and the US. Dr Coffey completed a NIHR Clinical Doctoral Fellowship in 2013 and a post-doctoral fellowship in 2017. She has published in leading peer-reviewed journals on the field.

CHAPTER 17

The Reality of Doctoral Project Management

Interview with Dr David Wilkie (Clinical Trial Manager)

1. Your doctoral research involved a lot of different studies and stakeholders. What did you need to deliver as part of your doctorate and what was the time frame you were given?

The purpose of my research was to investigate the role of information in therapeutic decision-making for adults living with multiple sclerosis (MS). At the time I was employed full time as a clinical trials manager specialising in MS, and my desire was to contribute to research in this field. Holding down a job meant I could only do my research part time, so I surmised that it would take me double the time required of a full-time student (around 6 years).

There were two milestone assessments at 18 months (9 for full-time students) and 36 months (18 if full time). The first review involved writing a detailed research plan incorporating a literature review and a presentation; the late-stage review was to present findings and data from the initial review and to determine if enough progress had been made for continuation. There were parallels to the initial review in terms of submitting a report and a presentation, but I had to show significant progress by this stage, and the initial research plan had to have evolved in the form of showing timelines to completion to potential chapter structure as part of the thesis.

It became evident that I was not going to meet the milestones, as the majority of my first year was dominated by my primary job as a trials manager. I therefore negotiated time away with my line manager and sought formal approval from the university to dedicate and split my working week between the PhD research and my main job. This ultimately added a year to the PhD timelines, but it was important to be clear with colleagues when I was not available and to have protected time to focus.

Working in the MS field gave me invaluable access to people living with the condition. At the time, I noticed that patients were sometimes struggling to come to a decision faced with a growing range of treatments with variable efficacy, risks and administrations. My initial aim was to determine patient priorities, and ultimately to direct support or even help to guide or influence treatment decisions.

2. As a doctoral student, did you receive any project management support, and what were the expectations?

In a broad sense, I would say that my experience of a PhD was that it was not at all like a masters or bachelors in the sense that I was not provided with a curriculum or a structured course to follow. By nature, a PhD is about discovering new knowledge, so there is often no road map. That said, there were university-led milestone, so the first year was defined by a literature review and determining trends as well as gaps in knowledge. Although the literature review is not limited to the first year – it is ongoing throughout the research – I never again had the time to dedicate to the literature and access to courses that I enjoyed in this first year. This was the point where I raised my base knowledge for what was to come.

Aside from this, my profession was advantageous in that I had experience of reviewing and executing trial protocols, so I was familiar with their structure. I also had experience of regulatory applications. This helped me to devise my own two studies without external support. I had deficits in my knowledge in other areas such as the statistical side of research, so this required more attention and learning. It really comes down to the individual to take charge and determine gaps in knowledge and how to fill them. I would encourage any doctoral students to utilise the resources offered by the institution and determine early on exactly what is expected in terms of study milestones and how the related documentation is to be structured and delivered.

Another area that was encouraged by my supervisor was to work on research papers in parallel with the PhD research. This proved invaluable, as the process helped me to structure content way ahead of the chapters that formed my thesis and to obtain independent peer review. I was also encouraged to enter and review my own data and to transcribe my own interviews with patients. It was time consuming but beneficial as I became familiar with the detail.

3. What approach did you use to ensure that you met supervisor expectations and delivered the projects on time?

I was employed as a clinical trials manager, which involved working as part of a clinical research team and conducting clinical trials across multiple hospital sites. This involved travel, so I had to learn to work on the move, and for this purpose I would utilise a laptop and workstations across sites. A portion of my PhD involved conducting a study involving questionnaire review and interviews, which meant I had to visit many clinics to approach potential subjects for involvement. This was very time consuming, and the clinics fell on set days and times of the week, so I had to be transparent with colleagues when I would be away and that there was the appropriate cover and oversight arranged in my absence, whilst maintaining project timelines as part of the portfolio of studies I helped to manage.

It is important to be open and honest about workload, as changes may need to be made in order to deliver the research. These changes may take the form of delegating tasks or requesting extensions as needed. There is no guarantee that the latter will be granted, but some components of a PhD can take longer than expected. There are certain life or world events (e.g. COVID!) that can't be mitigated in advance, but regular dialogue and communication with supervisors and involved colleagues can help to ensure that everyone is on the same page and working towards a common goal. I can only speak for my own university here, but I would expect there to be equivalents elsewhere. Ideally there will be a detailed handbook that outlines what is offered by the institution, from counselling to financial support, referencing, plagiarism guidelines and more. There should be clear guidance on who to approach for specific or specialist advice, and the general timelines and expectations of the degree you are conducting. There may also be variations of requirements depending on the faculty in which you are conducting the research.

4. In terms of project management, were there any strategies, tools or resources that you found useful?

I think it is very helpful to be friends with people who are also on the PhD journey or who have completed it previously. Understandably it can be challenging for some people to understand if they are outside of it, and there may be weekends you can't make or appointments you have to cancel in order to meet a deadline or obtain the data you need. There will be times like that, but I would say it is very important to pencil in "me time" where you can indulge your own interests away from the PhD – for example, I volunteered outside of work, learned how to build a website and attended meditation classes (I also taught some classes for a period). For exercise I would go out jogging, particularly along the river Thames which I was lucky to live close to. I would take advantage of living in London by visiting galleries and parks at weekends (it's surprising how much of it is free). If I had spare time at weekends, I would often take a random bus or, on a whim, take a train to nearby towns and cities to explore. The change of environment was important not just personally, in the sense that I was socialising and being reminded that there was life beyond work and research, but creatively it is important to give your mind the room to breathe. I found the environment I worked in could be less than inspiring, so the so-called "down" time was anything but. To illustrate the point of how important down time is, I actually came up with the first figure of my PhD whilst walking alongside a canal!

5. **On reflection, was there anything that you would have done differently considering your vast project and trial management experience to date?**
To a certain extent, the PhD is more about the journey than the outcome. It is very much a marathon rather than a sprint, so time management is crucial, but that is more challenging if you are years away from the outcome or can't quite grasp a concept. Looking back, even the u-turns were not failures. A study protocol is an academic proposal, so it may not work out in real-world terms. But you can make an amendment and try again. There is value in what you have changed. Small wins add up. One of the main issues with a PhD is staying motivated over a long period so just as important (if not more so than what software to use and how to manage time) are mental and physical health. It is easier to face the challenges of a PhD and stay motivated if you have this foundation. Approaching a PhD is as much off campus as on.

6. **Since your doctorate, you have managed a lot of larger, international studies. For those, does project management change, or do the same rules apply?**
Time management and being organised are pivotal in the execution of studies, particularly when sites are geographically dispersed and staff are in different time zones. I did not have this concern when I did my PhD, as the research was conducted entirely in the UK, but there are trends in how research is conducted and delivered.

7. **Regarding project management, is there anything that you learned during your doctorate that you still continue to do to this day?**
There are general approaches to my everyday work that are informed by the PhD experience. Examples include being able to read long documents efficiently and editing down content. Having an instinct for what is priority is critical.

8. **In your experience, what are the key determinants of project failure?**
Failure to adapt. Repeating past mistakes and being stubborn or rigid in your approach to tasks. If something doesn't work time and time again, then learn from it, switch and adapt.

Ineffective time management. Every day was precious during a PhD, but that does not mean every day is relentlessly worked. There will be times when a "down" day is useful to recover and regroup, so it's not all about racking up the hours in the office or in the lab, but instead the quality of the time you have versus the quantity. Of course you have a finite amount of hours to deliver it all, but chunk up the time wisely, determine when you are most efficient and make your calendar work for you.

9. **How do you sense when something is failing and how do you control for this?**
Failure is open to interpretation, and there is still value in finding out what doesn't work. The key is not to keep repeating it but to learn from it. I think there is a confidence you can gain from conducting your own mitigation strategy. It's like performing an audit once in a while. This can take the form of organising your data better so it is accessible and works for you. Also remember to back it up in case something goes wrong and have a system in place where you are always accessing the correct or most current database. Keeping a record of your data across its versions helps, as this creates a narrative. Notetaking is also useful but only if you can understand the content and make sense of it later. Although some things are out of your control, knowing you can implement a Plan B or C if Plan A fails definitely helps.

10. What are your top three project management tips?

1. Prepare to fail. In some ways it will be the failures or missteps that decide the direction of your project. If you accept early on that there will be experiments that don't work out but you can learn from the experience, then you have already prepared yourself mentally for what is to come and how to use it in the best possible way to inform your next move.

2. Communicate. This takes several forms, but first of all I would get used to writing and presenting your material whenever the opportunity arises. Ultimately the thesis is telling a story, so the more familiar you are with the narrative and how best to communicate this to the audience, the more confidence you will have in interpreting and conveying what you have learned.

   Effective communication also takes the form of making the most of the people around you and reaching out to them if needed. If you are struggling or have frustrations or just need to talk through where to go next with your project, having meaningful relationships – both personal and professional – can help to support and direct you.

3. Mitigate. A PhD might not come with a template or instructions to follow, but you can create your own road map based upon your best assumptions at any given time. On this road map you can even plot a few detours. If you plot out where you are headed, it can make you see the small parts and how they fit into the bigger picture. It might be that you have to u-turn or use a side road a few times on the journey, but if you have already planned for it, it will come as less of a surprise and instil a sense of confidence and direction not just in yourself but in those who are part of the journey, such as supervisors. This can take the form of mapping out your day on the day, but also a broader, high-level calendar which has milestones you must meet as part of the university requirements as well as project aims.

Dr David Wilkie is an experienced clinical trials manager of both national and international clinical trials. In 2020, Dr Wilkie was awarded a PhD from Imperial College London for his research aiming to support decision-making for patients with multiple sclerosis. He undertook his PhD alongside his clinical trials manager role at Imperial College, where he managed large multiple sclerosis trials at site level. Given the extent of his experience, he was subsequently employed as a global clinical trial manager contracted to Amgen, and a senior country coordinator at Marken. Dr Wilkie is currently employed as a study lead by Allergy Therapeutics, an international biotechnology company, where he leads a first-in-human study being conducted in the US.

CHAPTER 18

Reflections From an Experienced Doctoral Supervisor and Mentor

Interview with Professor Lisa Roberts (Musculoskeletal Physiotherapy)

1. **In your opinion, what are the key differences between supervision and mentorship?**
   Supervision is usually focussed on a task, such as completing a research dissertation, or undertaking a higher degree. Meanwhile, mentoring is more about helping you to reach your potential and often involves someone sharing their experience to help you progress. This can involve helping you to decide about career decisions, how to approach challenging situations in your role, by providing the opportunity to discuss them with someone outside of your team (or organisation), and so they can focus on helping you to decide what is best for you (rather than your service). Generally, supervision happens more frequently (and will differ if you are studying full or part time) than mentorship (which is often quarterly, to give you time to think and progress your plans).

2. **During the doctoral process what should healthcare professionals expect from their supervision experience?**
   The relationship with your supervisors is a special one! Firstly, there should be regular sessions of protected time in which you discuss your ideas and plans with your supervisors, and they help you to focus and clarify your thoughts. It may be helpful to think of this process as a car journey! You are in the driving seat, and you have set the destination in your satnav (completing your PhD). Your supervisors will help you to find the best route, help to prevent you going down too many dead ends (or driving off a cliff!) and will be there to support you as you travel this new route. If needed, they can help you to get back on track if you experience any untoward hazards along the way! This is completely different from being employed in a research post where you are an assistant on your supervisors' project. In doctoral work, you are required to produce an original contribution to the evidence base, and so you will be in the driving seat. It's like learning to drive, when at first it may feel a bit unnatural, with lots of things to master, but with practice and experience, the ride will be smoother!

   Supervision sessions should be fun, engaging; at times they are intellectually challenging, and above all should be positive and constructive. To get the most out of them, you need to plan your session carefully and manage your supervisors. What do you want to get out of the session? It is a time to share what has gone well and what you are struggling with, so that your supervisors can suggest some resources or ideas to help you move forward. They want (and need) to hear about the good, the bad and the ugly!

3. **What expectations do supervisors have of their students?**
   As a supervisor, I expect students to be organised – to plan sessions well in advance and come to the sessions with an account of what they have been doing, where they are at and what help they would like. We agree upon appropriate timescales for looking at work and providing feedback, and wherever possible, we discuss feedback together, either in person or online. I am not expecting them to come with everything sorted – right from the outset, we agree to share the highs and the

lows, and to remember that asking for help is a sign of strength, not weakness. I expect students to be honest, to flag up if they are finding something hard, but above all I want them to have a positive experience and enjoy their unique journey. After all, they are the supervisors of the future!

4. Is it possible for doctoral students to select their doctoral supervisor(s)?

Sometimes. It is usual to have two supervisors for doctoral studies, although sometimes there can be three to ensure that you will have the help you need with the topic and the methodology that you are planning to use. It may be that the PhD is set up as a project fellowship that the supervisor has gained funding for, in which case the funding is linked to the supervisory team, and so there won't be the option of choosing your supervisor. If you are applying for a personal fellowship (through a funding body such as the National Institute for Health Research), there is more scope to choose your supervisor and university. Sometimes it can be tricky if supervisors are in different universities, as both institutions would like a share of the doctoral fees. What is important in making these choices is to ensure that the university you are planning to apply to has all the support you need in terms of people and infrastructure.

5. What happens if you do not get on with your supervisor? Is there anything that you can or should do in this case?

In each university, there is a doctoral college or equivalent where there is a director who oversees all doctoral students. If you have any concerns or feel it is not working with your supervisor, it is really important to raise these concerns early, with your supervisor if you are able to or, if not, with the doctoral college. They will help you to find a solution, which may involve having a supported discussion to see if the problems can be solved, and if not, they will help you to find a different supervisor.

6. Why are mentors important during the doctoral journey?

Mentors are important because they focus on you rather than your research. They are there to share their experience and insight, to help you think about your career, role, plans for the future, etc. They do not get involved in discussing the detail of your research (that is the role of the supervisor). They are particularly important when you are facing times of change – for example, what are you going to do at the end of your doctoral studies, and how do you make these plans happen?

7. How do you recommend finding a suitable mentor?

Some organisations, such as NHS Trusts, have their own mentorship schemes, either as stand-alone opportunities or as part of a leadership course. Sometimes professional bodies offer mentorship too. There are also schemes through funding bodies, such as the National Institute for Health Research, which may help you to find an appropriate mentor. It is helpful to think about what aspect of your world you would most like help with. If it is career development, you may want to think about someone who has the sort of role that you aspire to: for example, if you would like to develop as a clinical academic, you may seek a mentor who has both academic and clinical roles. They do not have to be from the same profession as yourself, or even from your own organisation. They may be someone you already know, or someone you have heard about or seen at a conference or professional event. When you approach them, be clear what you are asking them to do – is it to potentially work with you as a mentor for the duration of your PhD, or is it to help you over the next 6 months as you plan to make some changes to your role?

8. How do you recommend preparing for doctoral supervision or mentorship meetings and how do they differ?

For both types of meetings, it is essential to think through before the session what you would like to focus on – an outline agenda. For supervision sessions, it may include a list of tasks or actions, whereas in mentoring sessions, it is often a particular problem or decision that you would like to discuss. It is helpful to discuss these at the start of the session, to set the agenda and ensure you cover what you wanted to in that session. If it is something you would like your supervisor/mentor to think about ahead of the session, you can negotiate with them to send some outline thoughts through, in an agreed-upon timescale. More often, the agenda is clarified at the start of the meeting.

9. **Do you remain in touch with any of your doctoral supervisors and mentors, and how important are/were they in your career success to date?**
It is important, especially in mentoring relationships, to agree at the outset how you would like to exit this phase. It may be that you work together for a particular time period, such as a year or two, or it may be for a particular task, such as completing your doctorate. You can then negotiate if you would like this to continue and if it is possible for your mentor. Likewise, when you finish your doctorate, it is good to have a plan about whether you would like to continue working with your supervisors as collaborators, if you are going on to apply for post-doctoral research fellowships, etc.

10. **What are your top three tips for doctoral supervision and mentorship success?**
   1. Choose your supervisors/mentors carefully. It is a special relationship, and you want someone who you are developing a positive relationship with, who will be there for you and can help you to achieve your goals.
   2. Take advantage of support sessions offered by the doctoral college, to meet with other students, to hear about their experiences and learn from them. Your journey will be unique, and this is a new experience, and so it is important to find out what others are doing and highlight any issues at the earliest opportunity. You will be managing your supervisors in this process!
   3. Remember that asking for help is a sign of strength, not weakness. After all, your supervisor/mentor has been where you are now and have found ways to make it work. As you navigate your route, they will be in the back seat, and are a great resource to help you succeed and fulfil your goals. Good luck!

Professor Lisa Roberts has a joint appointment as Clinical Professor of Musculoskeletal Health at the University of Southampton and Consultant Physiotherapist at University Hospital Southampton NHS Foundation Trust. The focus of her academic and clinical work is promoting musculoskeletal health, and her research priorities include: communication and decision-making; improving patient experience; promoting independence using web-based technologies; and advanced physiotherapy practice. Lisa has served on three national funding councils, published widely, is a former president of the Society of Back Pain Research, has multiple roles in Eurospine, and was a member of the World Health Organization Peer Review Group for Musculoskeletal Conditions. She is passionate about supporting and promoting clinical academic careers, has supervised 35 master's and doctoral students, and is a clinical academic mentor.

CHAPTER 19

Doctoral Development and Career Planning

Interview with Dr Kylie Watson (Midwifery)

1. **As part of your doctorate, did you have a personal development plan?**

   My successful application to the NIHR included details not just about the project that I was planning on doing but about how I would develop clinically and professionally over the course of the PhD. For me, this included training on specific research methods that I would be using to undertake the research, such as qualitative interview skills, mixed methods training and systematic reviewing. The first year of my doctorate was spent undertaking a number of master's in clinical research papers, and the subsequent years included development was undertaken at specific time periods in my study to align with when I would be doing different parts of the research. The university also had a very good doctoral academy, which provided excellent training and development sessions on ethics, literature searching and academic writing. It was also important for me to think of other development along the way, and this included undertaking a senior leadership in healthcare programme towards the end of my PhD.

2. **How did you identify the areas that you needed to develop, and were there any resources that you found helpful?**

   It was thinking about the skills that I would need and then finding the right resources for that. That funding was included for this in the PhD was hugely helpful and meant that I could be creative about the courses and programmes that I did. My supervisors were also helpful in suggesting different training and development that I might want to consider. It was also helpful looking at a research development framework (e.g. the Vitae Researcher Development Framework) to identify skills that might be needed.

3. **Did your development requirements change through the doctoral process?**

   They probably did change over the course of the doctorate, where more practical research skills were undertaken in the beginning and then more advanced development towards the end.

4. **As a healthcare professional in research, did you have any transferrable skills that helped you with this process?**

   I had a lot of clinical experience prior to starting a doctorate and had also had some small research secondments that had whetted my appetite for doing a larger piece of work. As healthcare professionals outside of medicine (including nurses, midwives and allied health professionals), one of the skills we are taught is critical reflection, and I think that has been a transferable skill that has helped with some of the process of undertaking a doctorate – both in an academic and in a personal sense.

5. **When did you begin thinking about your post-doctoral career and why was this important?**

   I started thinking about my post-doctoral career before I started a doctorate. It was really important to me to remain in a clinical role in some way after undertaking a PhD, and so being a consultant midwife was the perfect fit. I had several discussions with senior midwives within my trust about this career plan and desire, so by the time I had completed a doctorate, I had a plan and a job opportunity. I work in a trust where clinical academic roles for healthcare professionals outside of medicine are valued and there is a clear career trajectory for staff wishing to work in this way.

6. **Did you have any mentors to help you?**

I did struggle a little bit with mentors along the way, and the mentor that I had allocated to me through one pathway didn't really work out. I think with mentors it is about finding someone that isn't in your supervisory team that you can bounce things off and get a different opinion from. I have close friends and family that work in research, so I think they became my mentors! I have a good mentor now, and that person is important in discussing my current career and research plans with.

7. **What role did your research supervisors play in career planning?**

My supervisors were very open to what I was planning careerwise, and one of them was very influential in ensuring that the role I went into after my doctorate was a true clinical–academic one with protected research time and an honorary university contract.

8. **Would you advise people to think ambitiously about their future research career?**

I think having a plan is very important, but that also needs to be flexible. There will be things that happen along the way that may make the road a bit more bendy, but if you have a destination in mind, then that helps. It is also crucial to keep having conversations with the people you might need to influence about your future career. And speak to other people doing what you want to be doing to find out what worked for them.

9. **Do you continue to evaluate your personal and career development to this day?**

I am constantly evaluating where I am and what I am doing! My post-doctoral phase has been challenging but very rewarding, and there are always people around willing to support and advise. For me it is now thinking about setting another goal and going for that!

10. **What are your top three tips for personal development and career planning success?**

   1. Try to think what you want to be doing in 5 years.
   2. Be creative in your personal development.
   3. Remember you are not alone on this journey.

Dr Kylie Watson holds a clinical academic role as consultant midwife at Saint Mary's Hospital, Manchester University NHS Foundation Trust, and is an honorary lecturer at the University of Manchester. She trained in New Zealand but has spent over 20 years working within many different clinical maternity settings within the United Kingdom. Watson completed a full-time NIHR PhD fellowship in 2019. Her clinical leadership roles are primarily focussed on midwifery-led care and pathways, including a midwifery-led birth after caesarean pathway. She also leads a large birth planning (including supporting women who wish to plan birth out with recommended guidelines) and postnatal listening service. Kylie's research interests have focussed on intrapartum care, including the use of wireless monitoring during labour. Current research is focussed on the maternity experiences of women living in areas of social deprivation and from Black, Asian and minority ethnic backgrounds.

CHAPTER 20

Health and Well-Being From the Perspective of a Doctoral Student

Interview with Meera Sharma (Radiography)

1. **Why did you decide to undertake a doctorate and how far are you into your doctoral experience?**

   I decided to embark on my doctorate because it felt like the next personal and career progression step forward. My decision to finalise my area of research was very difficult, as I enjoyed both education and healthcare areas. The support and encouragement from senior management, research-active colleagues and the programme director were instrumental in taking the brave step forward. I started my journey prior to the COVID-19 pandemic and took some time away from my studies due to unforeseen personal circumstances. I have passed the first formal assessment for doctorate registration and am now continuing to the next phase of fieldwork and write-up.

2. **In terms of health and well-being, what have you discovered so far?**

   At the initial phase of my doctoral study, health and well-being were not central to my learning journey. The focus was on doctoral goals and progress in my research discussions. My health deteriorated significantly while trying to balance and manage my career and personal goals. As an ethnic minority, feeling privileged to embark on my research journey, I was not brave to speak up when I encountered hurdles that led to the feeling of being helpless during my studies earlier on. I found it difficult to speak up for help, as I was not sure of what kind of support was available. It was not until the COVID-19 pandemic that I decided to connect with the wider research and AHP community.

3. **What have you learned from your peers, mentors and supervisors in this regard?**

   The learning journey from peers undertaking a doctorate has been valuable for vulnerable conversations to discuss experiences and share information. This led to a better understanding that I am not the only one experiencing isolation or struggling in certain aspects of my doctorate.

   Mentors are critical for learning and providing insight into the research world. They give me a reality check into what it is like having research as part of their job plan or responsibilities.

   My supervisors are amazing, providing feedback and direction with my doctoral thesis. The relationship I have with them has led to confidence and self-belief that I can reach the finishing line.

4. **Are there any transferrable skills or approaches that you have found useful since transitioning from full-time clinical work to a clinical academic career?**

   There are many transferable skills such as time management, people interactions, communication skills with participants and supervisors, presentation skills, record keeping and tracking your ongoing work.

5. **Describe your 'go to' support systems during times of health and well-being challenge?**

   My 'go to' support systems during times of health and well-being challenge depend on what I need to face to move forward. My initial reaction now is to step away and enjoy a run or walk to bring focus. Thereafter I chat with my peers or post a note on the doctorate group about my issues for a solution. My final resort would be to have a conversation with my supervisors. The open conversations with my supervisors allowed me to continue with my studies when I faced personal and professional issues that impacted my study.

6. **Does your university provide health and well-being support, and how can you access this if you need it?**
I am not sure if or what kind of health and well-being support is offered to doctoral students. If suitable, I would access it in person and remotely. I have accessed alternative long-term support to help focus and balance my career development – an incredibly helpful career coach!

7. **What has been the biggest challenge to your health and well-being so far and how have you managed it?**
My biggest challenge to my health and well-being has been my mental health, caused by stress and worry about completing my doctorate successfully. The pressures of research impact and timely publications from the research world for ownership and recognition are high. As an ethnic minority woman, at times I have imposter syndrome traits or feeling that I am not good enough or thinking maybe I do not belong here. My long-term plan to manage this at present is having discussions with a career coach where I can be vulnerable and open in a safe space.

I had to make some drastic life-changing interventions to survive, as at one point I was struggling to balance family and studies during the COVID-19 pandemic. During the lockdown period, my husband's health was critical, and home-schooling responsibilities with no accessible support, including extended family, led to a reality awakening! It was the first time I started opening up and sharing my feelings and experiences with my supervisors and colleagues about my health and well-being, including my struggles. I learned to talk and trust key people, which changed my perception and helped my mental health. I also indulge in some chocolate and a good cup of coffee as my immediate go-to on some days! Self-care is central to my everyday living – exercise and eating healthy.

The small interventions led to looking at life differently and finding my happy zone or zen to survive and overcome challenges.

8. **What is the best way that you have found to wind down after a busy doctoral day?**
The best way for me to wind down is by going for a walk or watching some television or getting some sleep. It depends on how tired I am and when I finish. Most of the time it is going to bed early, as I am brain tired!

9. **As a doctoral student, how do you arrange a day off, what do you do and why is this important to you?**
I commit to my doctorate on a set day every week and I study small areas of my doctorate before starting or after work, such as correcting my thesis or reading a journal. I found if I left my studies to the dedicated day off, the first few hours I was always trying to figure out my next steps.

10. **What are your top three tips for looking after your health and well-being during the doctoral process?**
   1. Talk to your supervisors for support and direction of access to health and well-being services. My supervisors have been incredibly supportive with my doctoral journey for both personal and research growth. Health and well-being awareness need to be central to doing doctoral study. Also, accessing health and well-being support needs to be normalised during doctoral study. Many have shared lived doctoral study experience normalising health deterioration, including mental health, as an expected doctoral study experience. It would be valuable to have appropriate and accessible health and well-being support initiatives for ethnic minority students' postgraduate studies to encourage ambitions without their facing consequences or drawbacks.

2. Network and join research and writing groups. Small conversations with other healthcare professional students or researchers have led to opportunities and awareness of resources or tools that were helpful.

3. Make self-care part of your routine; the small daily enjoyable moments help to make the doctoral study journey feel less daunting!

Meera Sharma works in dual clinical and academic settings. In her current roles, she caters for the duality in the needs of both students and professionals within the healthcare system, which is very exciting, as it allows growth and application in both settings, which are continuously evolving. Meera has had many years of experience as a lecturer to develop as a leading educator, where she has had responsibilities with radiography programme deliverables at undergraduate and postgraduate levels. Meera is a doctoral student, focussing on lung cancer patients and caregiver experiences with diagnosis (medical imaging) and treatment (radiotherapy) for African Caribbean communities. Her additional research projects include AHP career decision-making, FAIResearch, career progression opportunities, workforce retention, career and upskilling the workforce to meet service demands.

CHAPTER 21

Experience of Being a Doctoral Parent

Interview with Dr Anthony Gilbert (Orthopaedic Physiotherapy)

1. **Undertaking a doctorate can be challenging as a parent/caregiver. How did you find it?**

   I found it easier during my PhD than I did during my MRes! For context, my youngest son was born in the first week of my MRes, and trying to write assignments with a 2-year-old hanging off me during the day and a newborn keeping me up at night was tough! I undertook my PhD 4 years later when my youngest was in his final year at nursery. Prior to having children, I hadn't really considered that there were difficulties with juggling work and home life. Being at home while I was working on my PhD was a privilege, as I got to spend more time around the family on a day-to-day basis. This wasn't always helpful, though—I recall many instances of paper writing being interrupted by 'Daddy, Daddy!' and the sound of metal cars running up the back of walls and doors to the humming of Disney Pixar's Cars soundtrack.

2. **Which specific challenges did you experience?**

   I am acutely aware that the challenges I faced are not unique to men – but I was able to take a break from clinical work as I undertook my MRes and PhD. These provided me with the time and space to undertake some of the work at home. During this time, I was exposed to the daily tasks that my partner did that, if I am honest, were previously invisible to me. As I reflect on my role in the household after my eldest was born, it was quite easy to slot back into my normal working pattern; I left for work early and got home for bath time 5 days a week and was hands on as much as possible during the weekends. When my youngest son was born, I was mostly working from home for the first few months of my MRes, as I needed to do a lot of coursework. I hadn't appreciated how much juggling went on. I read Arlie Hochschild's The Second Shift, and this helped illuminate some of these things for me. I think I stepped up and helped out a lot more during these times, but ultimately the MRes and the PhD were always competing with home life, which led to very little downtime!

   If I think specifically about the PhD work, it was always challenging being present in the household while trying to work. As much as I tried to set boundaries with the children, such as asking them not to come into my study when I was working or on a meeting, they just always seemed to want to be around me! Of course, I can appreciate how lovely this is, and I learnt to tune out background noise quite effectively. I became a regular customer at a local soft-play and often worked there at weekends while the children climbed the apparatus and hurtled down slides. As a PhD parent I became guilty of not being able to focus 100% of the time on my work (because of distractions from the children) or 100% of the time on my family (because of the PhD). There was always something else to think about, and I found this quite stressful. When the children were ill, I cared for them, and the PhD was put to one side. Previously, all the emergency caregivers' leave was managed by my partner. Being more present at home gave me the opportunity to support with some of these things.

I don't think I was an ignorant father or partner, but being at home during my PhD and MRes with young children did give me a much greater appreciation of the work that goes into running a household. I did experience the continual guilt of not being a good enough parent or partner (when I was doing the PhD work) or not being a good enough student (when I was being a parent or partner). I was guilty of not ring-fencing protected time for both. Until I learnt to do this, both suffered.

3. Can you describe any support or resources that you found most helpful?
I had several sources of support! I am someone who needs to talk through issues and challenges – I am not able to problem-solve as effectively in my head, and I developed a great MRes and PhD friendship group. We scheduled regular coffee meetups on campus or phone calls if we were on site; this is so important! I became a big fan of lunchtime walk and talks. Although wider doctoral groups are useful to get access to information, I personally prefer to speak more in-depth with trusted friends and colleagues.

At home, we always had a strict routine where the kids were in bed by 7 pm. This meant my partner and I always had the evening together. I am a big fan of cooking (and eating), and we made sure we spent this time together. I often returned to work later on after dinner, but it really helped to make sure we ate together and connected in the evenings.

While we did try online shopping, I actually quite enjoy going to the shops (and picking up my own PhD snacks), so it was always good to have the distraction of nipping out to the local supermarket for 30 minutes or so during the day.

4. Due to the pressures that parent/caring responsibilities inevitably pose, there are times when people may be tempted to quit. Did you ever feel like this and how did you keep going?
I didn't ever feel tempted to quit. I was very fortunate that my PhD was funded and I didn't have the financial pressure often faced by others. This privileged position enabled me to enjoy the process more than if I was worried about the financial aspects of a PhD. Undertaking a PhD without these pressures provided me with the opportunity to be present at home, and I was more connected with my family as a result. I am now in a job where I often work from home, and one of my favourite times of the day is when the children come home from school in the afternoon. I fear I would have missed out on that had I not undertaken my PhD when the kids were so young.

5. How did you balance clinical, research and family life? Which strategies worked best?
As a PhD student, I think I became the master of spinning plates. I worked in libraries, cafes, soft play, home, at the hospital … everywhere! The family calendar was an obvious necessity to plan family life, and I would make it clear when I would be away, which allowed my partner to plan. I would plan my day around the school run – this took some of the burden off my partner, who was then able to focus on her work. I made the time up in the evenings or weekends. I didn't put pressure on myself to stick to a 9–5 schedule; I was flexible, and this enabled me to enjoy and be good at both roles as a PhD student and member of the family.

6. Now that you have successfully completed your doctorate, is there anything that you would have done differently in terms of managing your time and energy?
I think I was very fortunate to have a trial run with my MRes, and I think I got the balance right with the PhD. I felt I was too rigid with my time while doing the MRes, which made things very tough for me to balance things with younger children. When I was more flexible and took breaks during the day to spend time with the kids, this served as a good opportunity to have a break from writing and blow off some steam. I would always make the time up later on in the evening, but I think I found the different working patterns difficult to adjust to after keeping to strict time schedules working clinically. I think some of my colleagues felt that I wasn't working if I wasn't being a clinician, and I felt some of that guilt for a while. I work best in blocks of 3 hours with a break if I am on a writing day, and there is nothing wrong with going for a walk or heading to the gym to break things up – I was always more productive after this. My advice to myself would be to

154

DOCTORATE: FINDING YOUR WAY

chill out and relax about the time of day I worked – as a PhD student you need space to think and a flexible approach to working patterns enables me to produce my best work.

7. In your current post-doctoral role, do you continue to employ these strategies, or have you needed to develop new ones?
I have fallen back into the NHS working pattern and I feel more guilt about taking time off during the middle of the day, so I don't really do that anymore. My boss encourages flexible working, so it is never a problem to take leave or adjust my working patterns for things like class assemblies. Now my kids are older and participate in a lot more clubs, I tend to do a lot of driving in the evenings; I don't have the energy to work late, so I am an early riser and try to get my work done much earlier now. It's now more of a challenge to schedule my annual leave across all the school holidays – this needs lots of planning ahead, as others in my team have children as well.

8. During my doctoral journey I experienced burnout as I learned how to manage the balance between work and family life. Did you ever experience burnout, and if so, how did it present?
I undertook my PhD during COVID, and I think everyone experienced burnout during this time, so I don't think I have any unique experiences on this. During my MRes I became quite unwell with a viral myocarditis which resulted from lots of work while caring for a newborn and training for a marathon. This forced me to rest. Naturally, I self-impose overly ambitious deadlines, and I have relaxed somewhat since that experience of being unwell. Thankfully, there are no long-term effects, but it was scary and was a good warning sign. There are certain triggers I can spot now: being tired, irritable, not being able to concentrate, overeating and drinking. I think I am better now at recognising when I need a break.

9. As a parent/caregiver in doctoral research, how did you overcome burnout?
I was very lucky to have a supportive team. As soon as I raised the fact that I was unwell with viral myocarditis, they supported me to slow down. Naturally I have quite an obsessive personality, and being given permission to not work myself to the ground was helpful! I'm much better at switching off now during annual leave. The COVID WhatsApp groups that were set up at the time were a great way to communicate, but I think they were actually quite damaging, as it made things difficult to switch off. I mute WhatsApp now and spend much less time on Twitter. I joined a golf club after my MRes and tried to play one or two times a month. Now as a post-doc, I am more involved in my children's sports and coach my youngest son's football team and help out at my elder son's swimming club. These probably bring new challenges in the context of family balance, but they serve as a great break from working life!

10. What are your top three tips for parents/caregivers undertaking a doctorate in healthcare research?
1. Do something at least once a week that you enjoy.
2. Don't set rigid timetables; do what works for you and your family.
3. Be kind to yourself!

Dr Anthony Gilbert has developed expertise as a clinical researcher over the last decade while working as a physiotherapist at the Royal National Orthopaedic Hospital (RNOH). Anthony completed an HEE/NIHR MRes in 2015 and was awarded his NIHR-funded PhD in 2022, which investigated patient preferences for remote consultations.
Anthony serves as an expert member on the London–Stanmore Health Research Authority NHS Ethics Committee. Anthony was the national chair of the Association of Trauma and Orthopaedic Chartered Physiotherapists (the Chartered Society of Physiotherapy Specialist Interest Group for orthopaedics and musculoskeletal care). He is the NIHR CRN North Thames Research Specialty Lead. In 2022, Anthony was awarded an NIHR Development and Skills Enhancement Award, where he is developing his knowledge and skills around clinical trials. He is an advocate for clinical academics and mentors several clinical researchers.

CHAPTER 22

Writing Your Way

Interview with Dr Marianne Coleman (Visual Science and Orthoptics)

1. Did you have any experience of academic writing before you started your doctorate?

Yes, I had already completed two publications in my professional body journal, supported by my university lecturers. I worked on these consecutively. The first one was developed from my undergraduate dissertation, so that was simply a case of reducing word count and deciding about the key messages for orthoptists. The second one was a brand new article idea suggested by my lecturers, about the differences in how certain orthoptic terms were defined and used in the academic literature and in practice. This required much more work, as I had a couple of starter terms suggested by the lecturers, but I then added a few ideas of my own, which each needed to be explored.

2. In your opinion, is it important to have had previous academic writing experience before you begin doctoral studies?

No, but it definitely helps. I think it is quite challenging as a clinician stepping into academia to have to get good at academic writing and designing clinical research projects all at the same time. There is also quite a big jump in expectations between undergraduate and masters/doctoral level writing as well. I learned this the hard way—I only scraped a pass on my literature review module for my master's in research degree, despite having two previous publications. My writeup was not good because I didn't go back to check that my introduction adequately reflected the results and discussion that came out of the review. What I said I was going to do in the intro did not reflect what I actually did! I was horrified when the marks came back, but it was an important lesson for me about the importance of revisiting sections to ensure the overarching narrative is maintained.

3. Which transferrable skills do we have as health care professionals to support our doctoral writing practice?

We're used to cramming our CPD whenever we can, so cram in your writing whenever you can too! If you are collecting data in hospital, write there. As healthcare professionals we do also have this ability to think outside the box in our practice, and this is also really applicable to the way that we write about research too. That's where innovation and novelty can come from. Also, a really important part of doctoral writing is communicating the purpose and benefit of our work, and as healthcare professionals our research is often grounded by these concepts as well, which puts us in a great place to explain complex research in a way that makes sense to the non-expert.

4. When did you begin writing your doctoral thesis?

Although I worked through the thesis chapters in the conventional way, starting with a literature review of the topic at hand to rationalise the work I was doing, I did not start writing as early as some others may have done. I actually spent the first half of my first year doing pilot studies and finishing off a relevant study from my master's degree, instead of starting my thesis. This actually was probably not ideal, as when I went to my first academic conference, I didn't get as much out of it as I could've done. If I had been reading papers to complete my first chapter, I think I would've gotten more out of the experience. In the end, I didn't complete the literature review chapter until the end of my first year. I think starting this earlier would have been better.

5. **How did you develop your writing skills during your doctorate?**
   I did attend some in-house writing courses, but honestly a lot of my scientific writing skills were already embedded from both my undergraduate dissertation, master's projects and from creative writing. I think it's important to read as well as write, because you have a much better sense of what is a good flow from reading good articles. I think your best writing comes from when you are in the flow, have a passion about the topic and you're enjoying what you're writing about. This is actually a psychological theory (flow theory), and it usually happens when you are in that coveted stage of having some degree of mastery about the topic (i.e. when you're doing most of your writing!). So I promise you that although the early stages of writing in your doctorate might be a bit torturous, you will get better at it the more you know your topic, and you will turn out some great work!

6. **Is it necessary to undertake external writing skills courses?**
   No. I didn't. It really depends on your own skills. If you think some professional coaching would really benefit you, then do what you need to do. But you know what can be helpful? Writing retreats! If your graduate school organises one, try and make it if you can. Having a different space to write and think in is always worth a try; you never know what it might do for you in terms of who you meet and what titbits you pick up from other people too!

7. **If someone has learning needs in this area, what would you recommend they do?**
   Every university has its own support procedures for graduate researchers. If English is your second language, there are usually services you can access to help you. If you need more specific support, ensure you reach out as early as possible so that your needs are appropriately documented and can be evidenced in any applications you make. Taking time out during a PhD is not uncommon and there is no shame in it if it's what you need to get back on track. However, try to write regularly, if you can manage it, as it can help with building up practice and feeling less overwhelmed. Ethics documentation for healthcare research is a great way to get started, as you usually need to supply some background to the research and be able to communicate your methods to a non-expert committee.

8. **How would you define 'writer's block'? Have you ever experienced it, and if so, how did you deal with it?**
   I think writer's block is more than just blank page syndrome. Constantly re-editing instead of writing new content counts as well! So does procrastinating looking stuff up and leaving a sentence half finished. I definitely have it on occasion. I make a lot of use of [] to fill in empty spots so I can then search for this later and fill it in properly. If you are able to, help your future self by writing something between those square brackets to describe what you're missing. It's an effective way to keep the momentum going without getting bogged down in "quick lookups" (they are never quick), but I have cursed my past self on multiple occasions for not putting enough info in between those square brackets to help me work out what I was thinking about at the time! Shut-Up-And-Write sessions with a buddy can be a great way to get through the writer's block too.

9. **How did you maintain your motivation to write throughout your doctorate? What worked and what did not?**
   Bribery! My partner instigated '1500-word Fridays' where he had a treat waiting for me at home if I had completed 1500 words (ish) that day. It was a good motivator for me to set aside writing time. Sometimes I wasn't in the mood for writing, but it was a good incentive to get something down on the page. Even if it's garbage, you can work with garbage. I just didn't want to miss out on a treat. What can I say, I am very treat-motivated!

Also, having the equipment to be able to write anywhere. As much as possible, work on the cloud and be portable. I wrote most of my thesis in a random clinic room at a local hospital while data collecting for my final study, which involved inviting families to drop by my computer at the end of their routine appointment. Twenty- to thirty-minute intervals are plenty long enough for a writing sprint!

10. What are your top three tips for writing success?
1. Accept that as a clinician researcher, you are rarely going to have dedicated writing time. Learn to make the most of those did-not-attends and random 20-minute writing slots to smash out a paragraph or two.
2. Try to make your first draft a good draft—it makes things much easier for your doctoral supervisor to focus their feedback on the really key things to make your work the best it can be.
3. Everyone has their own writing tips, and you need to find out what works for you! Not everything works for everyone, so try out different things and see what is best for you.

Dr Marianne Coleman qualified as an orthoptist in 2008 from the University of Liverpool. After some time in clinical practice, diagnosing and managing binocular vision and ocular motility disorders in children and adults, she completed a master's in research at the University of Liverpool and moved to Glasgow Caledonian University to study visual distortions arising in amblyopia for her PhD.

After completing her PhD, which was strongly focussed on clinical research, she coordinated the first UK randomised controlled trial evaluating video-game-based perceptual learning as a treatment for children with amblyopia. She moved to the University of Surrey in June 2016 to train in health services research, maintaining her clinical orthoptic research through funded projects evaluating binocular vision in skilled video game players and people living with dementia. Marianne has recently commenced a joint post as a clinical vision research fellow, working between the Department of Optometry and Vision Sciences and the Australian College of Optometry's National Vision Research Institute.

CHAPTER 23

Writing a Doctoral Thesis From the Perspective of an Experienced Examiner

Interview with Professor Chris Nestor (Podiatry)

1. **What is a thesis and why is it important?**

    Let's demystify a little and be less emotional about 'the thesis'. It is, first and foremost, only a vehicle for demonstrating how you meet the requirements for the doctoral (or other) award and setting your stall out for your contribution to a specific area of work. It is not a personal journal of the last 3 to 7 years of work that needs to map every idea, thought or activity you did. Nor is it a window into your life and all the pain doing a PhD has involved. It is your assignment report, no more and no less. See it as that and it will make writing it and moving on from the PhD a lot easier.

    Let's also remember that producing a thesis and doing a PhD is a human experience that is very emotional, so let's also try and embrace that in as much as it adds value and is good for you to do so. It's the first time you really put down a marker for what research looks like in your style and voice. There are many common features to all PhDs, and other theses, but there should also be space for it to reflect you too.

    Please don't look too hard for a thesis formula or jump to the first one you see. Theses are frequently non-linear in their content, so don't assume one chapter needs to build on the previous one in a stepwise fashion. The ideas you are dealing with are likely complex, and so you can expect the thesis structure and content to reflect this. It is fine to have chapters that might not directly flow on from the previous one, but you must show coherence across the entirety of the thesis. Part of the skill you need to show is your ability to communicate complex ideas and concepts coherently. The structure and the way you connect the chapters together to assist the reader is important alongside the content of each chapter. Think about the start and end sections in each chapter: Can you refer back or forward to other chapters in these parts to weave interconnections purposefully? This can make it easy for the reader to see both the detail in each chapter alongside a 'view from the helicopter' and therefore the entirety of your work. Both matter to examiners, and too often only the detail and chapter content matter to candidates.

2. **Did you enjoy writing your thesis?**

    I love writing and the process of crafting an argument, a case, drawing in evidence and appraising alternative views to take a reader towards a coherent conclusion. I start knowing there will be many iterations of the work, trusting the process and only looking that after a period of effort I am going in the right direction. I don't try to get too much polished before moving on to the next part. You learn through the process of writing, and so it is to be expected that you go back and forth between sections that have already been written, to adjust them and fine-tune in respect of the other parts you are still writing.

But I always have one piece of advice: don't use writing to work out what you want to say; use it to communicate what you want to say. So, you must spend time first planning the messages you want to convey. What order do they come in? What evidence or information will you draw upon to evidence each point you make? Please, plan plan plan, and only write once you are ready to communicate. Even then, expect many iterations. But really try and avoid writing for the purposes of discovering what to say – it is slow, painful and ultimately makes achieving quality more difficult.

Even try and plan the flow of your writing down the content of paragraphs. Try:

- The main message in paragraph x is...
- Say why is this message is to be believed using evidence, data, or other material.
- Say why this message is important and what the implications of it are, including for whom.
- Do you need to connect what you have said above to the next paragraph?

3. Is it important to read doctoral theses before writing you own?

Yes, but never read just one; browse many to give you comfort in the fact there is more than one way of writing a thesis successfully. Do read those in your field but never just those from your university. Departments and disciplines, especially at specific institutions, can fall into a pattern of types of theses, and if you are not careful, you won't learn about alternatives. Your supervisor might learn something too (yes, I said it, we don't have all the answers, and if we think we do, change supervisors).

I learnt the most about diversity in types of theses by acting as an independent chair for PhD examinations in disciplines such as music, English literature and the built environment, to name a few. Understanding how meeting doctoral criteria can be achieved in many diverse ways really prevents us from falling into poor habits and being reliant on rather tired models of theses. It also invites exploration of how, since we are expanding knowledge, the formats by which we communicate knowledge need to adapt. Theses need to reflect what you have done, not dictate it: make it your servant, not your master. Honour your work and the knowledge created, not the expectations of just your supervisor or department or discipline; otherwise, are you really acting as an independent researcher?

4. How can students access doctoral theses?

Most universities have open digital repositories of theses and I would look at several from your country, but also other countries where your discipline is research-active. I have examined PhDs from Singapore, Australia, Spain and Scandinavia too. There are important interpretations of how knowledge is created and presented for a PhD defence. Developing a wider appreciation helps to assure you there is no right and wrong way to curate your thesis, but there are consistent patterns to how they are drawn together. The most coherent thread across countries is:

- Clearly articulate reasoning for why the research is necessary.
- Use literature and policy contexts to precisely locate your work in the existing knowledge base.
- Present a clear methodology.
- Offer rigorous presentation and interrogation of data.
- Draw together what has been learnt and contextualise it within the wider discipline.
- Distil out key messages for your priority audiences.
- Be reflective on your work, the research questions and research delivery, your development as a researcher, and then look forwards to the future too.

5. At which stage in the doctoral process should students begin to write a thesis?

Writing takes time to get good. Start early but focus on short, manageable pieces of work. Your doctoral milestones or other assessments (e.g. end-of-year assessments) will provide a platform for this. It will challenge you to write about a lot of effort on your part but without a lot of words. Being concise is an important skill. You will practise and define the story of your PhD so that it can be captured in a sentence, or two at most. You will feel this short-changes you, does not reflect your hard work and fails to show everything you have learnt. But that is the reality of research: much goes on in the background, but what you need to show is only what matters to others, not what matters to you. Writing for dissemination (or assessment) is about meeting the needs of others in your field and discipline to help it forward in constructive and responsible ways. It is not about satisfying your need to have your work and deeds seen.

6. **What resources are currently available to students who find academic writing challenging?**
You are never alone. Speak to peers, join or set up a writing club, draw in experienced publishers/colleagues who have a responsibility to help develop writing as a critical academic skill. Do not fester away writing on your own.

   Protect time to write but equally learn to put it down. Forcing yourself to write for 2 or 3 hours can be unproductive, and yet a well-timed 30 minutes can produce wonders. So timely writing (i.e. when you have what you want to communicate well organised) is key, not just time writing.

   When you have written something you are pleased with, go back to your first version and track your progress; the difference and the reasons for the improvements will be stark, and it is an easy way to learn.

   Try to publish something, however minor or incremental – I certainly did this. My first few papers were small pieces of work and were really about enabling me to practise writing, receive peer review, evolve and learn from it.

   Expect some uncomfortable feedback. Journal reviewers in particular often do not take enough care to understand the author and where they might be in their career/journey. Too often they hold very hard to high standards and can be harsh without offering constructive advice with equivalent gusto. Be prepared for that (and try and not repeat it when you offer reviews).

7. **What expectations do examiners have when examining a thesis?**
When I receive a thesis, I know the candidate has been through several prior internal assessments; supervisors have seen, read and fed back on the thesis too. So there is an implicit expectation that it is likely fit for purpose and will pass. But I always hold firmly the option to fail and I have been involved in two PhD fails and several master's in research failures too. Without exception, the reasons for failure lie way back in the PhD journey and are not about the thesis. Often the candidate and the supervision team have lost trust in each other and become dysfunctional; often the candidate is not responding to advice. Too often candidates have been too pragmatic in their decision-making, have rushed and not relied on academic process and reasoning for the research decisions they have made, and so their PhD narrative unravels when they try to write it up as a coherent piece of work. The examiners will quickly see through it.

   I want to see a deep appreciation of the literature and especially of research that is very close to the research problem being addressed. I want to see both a gap in knowledge defined and a case for why filling that knowledge gap is worthwhile. Remember that just because something has not been done before is not a reason to do it. Indeed, there could be very good reasons that no one has researched X or Y before; maybe it is futile to try, or the knowledge gained would be so incremental, it's not worth the effort (at least not for a doctoral award).

   Examiners will often look for why something was done far more than candidates realise. We are not just interested in what was done. We want to see your intellectual skills alongside any practical research delivery skills. If you deliver a research study but without intellectual reasoning, you are a researcher worker, following the designs and directions of others. That is not the independent researcher we want to see for a PhD award. Where is the novel research question you defined, and why is that question important? What are the possible research designs that could help answer that question, and why did you choose the one you did?

   We also don't, I hope, expect a candidate to do only what we would have done. I am happy to disagree with a candidate if they have a reason to think differently than me. So please don't feel compelled to write to please the examiner, be more confident and clear in your position, but in doing so always consider the views of others alongside your view. Rarely is there only one answer to a research question, or research design or approach to data analysis that could be pertinent. Choose your path but recognise the value in the different options that other people hold too.

8. Can a thesis be used to support performance at a viva voce examination?

Absolutely – in fact, I want to see a candidate (and advise my own students) to physically use their thesis in the viva. If a question comes up and the answer is already in the thesis, say so, and show so: go to the page, turn the thesis around and invite the examiner to see it (or they will just ask for a page number and look at their own copy). This can be especially useful if your data help to answer the question – take the examiner to the data plot, diagram or figure and explain how what is shown answers their question. This shows you know the thesis, own the contents and understand how to use it too, all hallmarks of a successful PhD defence.

I always advise my students to plan/practice answers to the topics that you know will come up. These might either be decisions that were made in the PhD where you know others might think differently, or where you had the most learning to do and might feel weak. Plan for these certainties (why would you not?).

- Be prepared to explain what you did versus what supervisors or other candidates/researchers you might have worked with did. Be clear on the specific intellectual contribution you made.
- Always do a fresh literature search a few days before and be prepared to bring into the viva literature that has been published since you submitted the thesis. It doesn't look good when an examiner does this on your behalf ('Have you seen this paper?' … and then you have not).
- If you have a list of your own corrections or things you want to change in the thesis, bring it with you and be able to talk through it.
- Be prepared to draw or use other means to argue your case, make a point or illustrate something. If an examiners asks, 'What would happen to this data if you did X or Y to your participants?' be prepared to use a number of different ways to answer – for example, draw hypothetical data on a chart and draw out how it might change if X or Y intervention were used, or show how a different statistical test might treat data differently. This can help to bring to life an idea that you may have found difficult to explain in words. It also helps to show your knowledge and confidence in using it in constructive dialogue.
- Remember, you are the expert on your work – the examiners do not know your journey and thesis as you do. You are the expert in your thesis. They are experts in the discipline you are working in and see your thesis only through that lens.

9. What is plagiarism and what should you do to avoid it?

One way to avoid plagiarism is to simply be clear about how you will use the work of others. If you took an idea from paper A, say so, and if you wish to propose a new idea, then make it clear how that idea relates to those of others. You could do this with a diagram, not just in writing.

Occasionally you come across a phrase that captures an idea so well you cannot imagine writing it any better – great! You can honour the achievement of others by simply using it word for word but in quotation marks. So, where you feel there is added value, directly quote people or papers, but be honest about it – this shows you recognise boundaries between scholars and wish to give full credit to sources, and helps to build a sense that everywhere else (where you do not do this), the work is yours.

Examiners will look for consistency in terminology between parts of the thesis and in the viva. Using different terms interchangeably or relying on lay rather than appropriate technical terms are red flags for not owning or understanding your work and an overreliance on the words of others. You say 'people do not need', but do you mean patients, participants, people in other parts of the healthcare system or people in the audience of your research? As you use these terms interchangeably, it matters. Be precise and also consistent.

If writing styles change, that is also a red flag for me. It is okay to have had more time to refine one chapter versus another; we can discuss that at the viva. But there is a difference between something being less polished and two chapters being in different styles – did you write them both, really? Does this mean you are trying out different writing styles? How would you describe your approach to writing your thesis? Or did you write one section before and another section after perfecting your writing or some training? Maybe one has been published as a journal paper, and therefore you have been able to benefit from extra peer review from outside your supervision team?

10. What are your top three tips for thesis submission success?

1. Have a whole thesis plan and actively discuss where the boundary of 'too much thesis' lies. I once heard a colleague say that he never wants to see a thesis of more than 150 pages, or the candidate is not being concise enough. I disagree with that limit, but I do think you need to be clear on why a thesis is a lot more than, say, 200 pages. If you cannot show you meet the doctoral criteria in 200 pages … then how many more pages do you need? Or are you trying to include too much work just because you did it whilst you were doing your PhD? Remember, the primary written currency of academia is publishing papers that are 3000 to 4000 words. Being concise is a skill worth practising. More is definitely not better in many cases.

2. Do not plan to go to the wire. Finish a week ahead of the deadline, leave time for files to crash … printing … (if you still need to do that), unforeseen errors and corrections you will need to make. No one escapes these issues, I promise you, so expect them.

3. Do set a firm deadline if you are not given one. You could go on forever making improvements, but at some point you will be making decisions and making changes that have no bearing on what the examiners will think. So hand it over and let them get on with their work. Do carry on checking it, however, and planning to correct/update it, but you will never be able to design out an examiner wanting to change something—so don't try.

Professor Chris Nester is a podiatrist by first degree and has published over 150 journal papers and had 23 PhD students complete their studies with him. His research uses quantitative and qualitative approaches to understand foot and lower limb health with work spanning public health, community and acute care contexts.

CHAPTER 24

The Viva Voce Is Your Time to Shine

Interview with Dr Donna Kennedy (Occupational Therapy)

1. How would you describe the day of your viva?

The day of one's viva is an exhilarating, albeit terrifying, milestone. My academic supervisors were well experienced in supporting PhD students, so I had a good understanding of what to expect on the day. I knew I would sit in a room across from two examiners, experts in their fields. They would ask me questions, exploring any and all aspects of my thesis. I've heard that at some universities, the supervisor sits with the candidate during the viva. Mine did not; this is not procedure at Imperial College, and I was glad for it. I was the independent scientist, defending my work, without my supervisor there to rescue me.

I'd been reminded by a supervisor that this might be the only time that two people would sit and listen to me discuss my work at length, so I should relish the opportunity. While I felt well prepared, I think it is only human to expect disaster to strike on such a momentous occasion. Your mind might go blank and you can't discuss your work. Or you are asked something you just can't answer.

My examination took place in the conference room of my group's offices. While I think others opt for a more neutral setting, I was pleased with this, as it felt like home to me after 3-plus years. I think the length of the viva varies by examiners and candidates and can be as brief as 1 hour. My viva lasted for 3 hours, and I was limp with fatigue and relief at the end of it.

2. How did you prepare? Is there a best way?

I'm not sure there is one right way to prepare for a viva; however, there seems to be agreement on many aspects of preparation. For the days leading up to the viva, I maintained my routine of daily exercise. I ate well and went to bed early enough to ensure a good night's sleep. I travelled by public transportation, so I allowed enough time to deal with potential delays. I arrived 1 hour early—enough time to get settled and get my head in the game, but not so much time as to get jittery. I wore professional but comfortable clothes. I wanted to wear something that made me feel confident but didn't want to be conscious of my clothing during the viva. I prepared my clothing the day before, so I wasn't fumbling with an iron on the day. On viva day, I brought a backup top in my bag should I do something silly like spill coffee on my blouse before the viva. I didn't want to start off in stains!

I brought the draft of my thesis but removed all the highlighted tabs that I'd been using to identify sections for review. I didn't want to highlight how many of these review areas there were, and figured I could rely on the table of contents if necessary. My viva began at 11:00. I'd had a good breakfast and then ate a protein-rich energy bar shortly before starting the viva. I brought water into the viva, but nothing else.

3. Did you find it helpful to discuss the viva voce process with experienced peers, mentors and/or supervisors?

I discussed the viva process with peers and supervisors in advance. It was helpful to consider my responses to questions, to appreciate what are seen as strengths and what might be interpreted as weaknesses. For example, I'd heard of a candidate who was unable to explore their own work critically and came across as defensive. To avoid this pitfall, I started most of my answers with "that's a great question, thank you!" and then proceeded to elaborate. I also reviewed my methods and analysis prior to the viva, and considered other ways I might have performed or analysed my work. This enabled me to discuss my choices and their relevant merits and weaknesses freely.

Prior to the viva, my supervisors advised that I get to know the academic work of my examiners. While this may seem obvious, I was so worried about my own work, I hadn't considered theirs! So I went through my examiners' grants and publications, and this allowed me to consider my work in the context of theirs. I think this may have made for a more interesting discussion on their part; it certainly enhanced the discussion for me.

The final tip I garnered from colleagues and supervisors was to stay abreast of the literature until the moment I walked in the room. During the viva, the candidate needs to discuss their work in the context of the current evidence in the field. If a relevant, earth-shattering discovery was published prior to the viva, a good scientist would know about it! So I continued to read the tables of contents for relevant journals, ensuring I was abreast of the emerging evidence.

4. How much did the doctoral process itself prepare you for the viva?

The viva is the culmination of the learning and growth that happens over the course of the doctoral fellowship. When I started my fellowship, I was so nervous I didn't want to get up to make a cup of tea. By the time I'd finished, I was organising corridor cricket contests (please don't report me to the health and safety team!). At the start of my fellowship, my supervisor told me that in the first year he would teach me, the second year he and I would learn together, and by the third year I would be teaching him. And this was certainly the case.

Participating in our group's journal clubs and team presentations sharpened my critical appraisal and debating skills. Working and learning with a diverse group of clinicians and academics encouraged me to take both a micro and a macro view to questions and plausible answers.

During my fellowship, I was required to complete early- and late-stage PhD reviews. These reviews were college requirements, and intended to ensure I was on track for completing my project per plan. I presented my work to date, but in writing and orally, to two academics outside of my supervisory team. The early- and late-stage reviewers examined my work, ensuring it was of sufficient quality and quantity to merit a PhD, while providing me with much needed reassurance that I was inching my way towards the goal.

Members of our group were encouraged to submit our work for publication and to international conferences. By the time I sat my viva, I had published a paper in a top journal and presented my work orally at multiple international conferences. These opportunities helped me to present my work clearly and to answer questions graciously and succinctly. By viva day, I had been living my work for years: presenting it, explaining it. I was definitely ready to defend it.

5. Did you have the option to select the external examiners or did your supervisory team select the external examiners for you?

I had one internal and one external examiner. My supervisors made suggestions regarding appropriate examiners, but they allowed me to have the final say on who would be asked. This was important to me. We all know in which environments we thrive and in which we wilt. I choose examiners whom I respected and admired but who didn't strike terror in my heart. I think I choose well.

6. **Some doctoral students choose to undertake a practice viva beforehand. Did you avail yourself of this opportunity? Did it help?**

I did a sort of pseudo-viva with my research group, presenting my work and answering questions. This was useful, as none were from the same clinical background as me. It's important to be able to explain your work clearly to those in other fields and disciplines. Sort of like a 60-minute elevator pitch! This definitely helped me to prepare for the big day. I also trawlled through websites and found lists of viva questions. I compiled them and ensured I would be prepared to answer such questions.

7. **On the day of your viva, when and how did they share the outcome with you?**

On the day of my viva, when the questions and answers were finished, my examiners adjourned to another room. I left the viva room, thoroughly exhausted after an intense 3-hour examination. I made a cup of tea and sent a message to my family that I was done. I was confident I had done enough to pass. The relief was immeasurable.

I'm not sure how long I waited for the news of my result. It was at least 30 minutes, but to be fair, it's a bit of a blur. My supervisor came to my desk and addressed me as Dr Kennedy. Hurrah! I was called into my supervisor's office to discuss the viva outcome with my supervisor and examiners. There are numerous possible viva outcomes, ranging from pass to not pass to fail. I passed, with minor amendments, and I'm told this is the most common result. In this situation, the candidate is requested to make a few minor corrections and submit them to the examiners within 3 months. Upon approval by the examiners, the degree is awarded. In other possible viva outcome scenarios, the candidate may have not passed but is allowed to rewrite the thesis or re-sit the viva in examination for a PhD. And finally, disastrously, some candidates may fail the viva. In these situations, the candidate may fail the PhD but have produced work adequate for an MPhil. Or the work may be deemed a fail, with no possibility of a degree. Thankfully, I would presume failure is a rare occurrence, given the thorough checks and balances that are in place to circumvent this result.

In addition to my viva outcome, my examiners shared a few additional details. They shared that they had very much enjoyed examining my work (perhaps they have to say that?). They found my thesis to be very well organised, and this made it easy to read and digest. And they enjoyed the discussion of my work and our interchange of ideas. It was wonderful to have positive affirmation after years of work, that my work was novel, innovative and important.

8. **How did you choose to celebrate?**

On the afternoon of my viva success, my supervisor treated me and one of my examiners (the other couldn't stay) to a late lunch at a local restaurant. I recall very little of the meal or conversation. I was ravenous, having not eaten since morning. I was physically exhausted from the mental strain of the examination. And I was ecstatically happy; I was a doctor! Over the coming weeks, I celebrated my success with family and friends. They were as delighted for me as I was for myself. At my very next teaching session, I was elated to change my title to Dr Kennedy. It is taking a long time to get used to the new title; I'm still not sure it has fully sunk in.

9. **What are your top three tips for viva voce success?**

1. Know your own work inside and out. It may sound strange, but you'll be discussing decisions you may have made 3 or 4 years earlier. Reacquaint yourself with the thread that runs through your work; be prepared to share your work with fascination.
2. The limelight is yours to shine in; remember that. Relish the opportunity to share and explore your work and ideas with experts. Receive your examiners questions with gratitude and curiosity. Enjoy this exchange of ideas.
3. Present your work, or at least elements of it, as often as you can prior to your viva. Practice sharing your work with diverse and maybe even hostile audiences (not everyone may welcome your results if they contradict their own!). Presenting and defending your work to various forums will strength your skills and prepare you for the big day.

Dr Donna Kennedy is a hand therapist and senior clinical academic for occupational therapy at Imperial College Healthcare NHS Trust (ICHT) and is an Imperial Clinical Academic Training Office (CATO) postdoctoral research fellow in the Pain Research Group, Department of Surgery & Cancer, Imperial College London (ICL). Donna completed a BSc in occupational therapy at Tufts University in 1984 and an MSc in health sciences from the University of East Anglia in 2009. Donna has extensive clinical experience with expertise in hand trauma and acquired, rheumatologic and surgical conditions of the hand and upper limb. Thirty years after completing her undergraduate training, she undertook a National Institute for Health Research (NIHR)-funded clinical doctoral research fellowship. Donna was successfully awarded a PhD in pain research from Imperial College London in 2018; she was the first allied health professional (AHP) to be so recognized.

CHAPTER 25

Celebrate Your Impact and Success

Interview with Professor Kerry Gaskin (Nursing)

1. **The doctoral journey is long, with few wins along the way. Which wins did you choose to celebrate?**

   There were several key milestones throughout the journey that were celebrated in different ways. At the beginning of the project, gaining funding and ethical approval were important achievements allowing us to implement the project and were personal high fives! Other personal milestones were completing data collection and analysis, completing and submitting my thesis, completing the viva and my graduation ceremony.

2. **Why was it important to you and your stakeholders to share and celebrate your successes?**

   It was important to disseminate the project findings through publications and conferences nationally and internationally, as we developed a novel early warning tool for parents of infants who had undergone complex cardiac surgery. There has been positive research impact for parents in terms of recognising clinical deterioration in their infants and timely and structured communication with health care professionals and appropriate management of the situation. Doing something important for families to help them keep their infants safe at home was a motivator for me throughout the doctoral journey.

3. **How did you typically celebrate and share your success during your doctorate?**

   Success was shared through social media (Twitter, LinkedIn, Facebook), publications in peer-reviewed journals and presenting the work nationally and internationally at research seminar series, conferences and family days held by the national congenital heart disease charity Little Hearts Matter. I was shortlisted for nurse scientist of the year in 2016 at the Children's Hospital of Philadelphia 19th Annual Update on Pediatric and Congenital Cardiovascular Disease Conference, at Loews Royal Pacific Resort at Universal Orlando Florida, and came a close second!

   My viva success was celebrated quietly with close family by going out for a meal. My graduation ceremony was the biggest and most special celebration, as it was also my grandma's 92nd birthday. I was lucky to be given three extra tickets into the cathedral, as a friend who was graduating didn't have any guests, so my partner, children, parents, and grandma were able to join me and had front row seats!

4. **As healthcare professionals, we typically struggle to celebrate our successes. For a new doctoral student who may be keen to share but does not know where to begin, what would you recommend?**

   I would recommend orally presenting the ongoing progress of work throughout the doctorate at smaller events such as showcasing your work at team, department or organisation events, as well as research seminar series and post-graduate conferences within the university. Look for relevant local, national or international conferences where you can present your work, grow your networks and learn from others in the same field. These are useful for testing out your ideas and developing confidence in your ability to defend the developing thesis. Another great way to disseminate progress is to have a logo developed for your project, set up a Twitter account for the project using the logo, create infographics and consider writing a blog with updates on progress.

5. **Can you describe any support or resources that you found most helpful when it came to sharing your research successes?**
As part of my doctoral research, I led the development of parental home monitoring and assessment of infants with complex congenital heart disease using an early warning tool called the Congenital Heart Assessment Tool (CHAT), to enable parents to identify signs of deterioration in their infant and to make prompt contact with the appropriate healthcare professional. I found online dissemination a good way to communicate the progress of the project. I set up a Twitter account @CHATool, and post-doctorally I created an e-learning resource for staff, which is freely available through the Congenital Cardiac Nurses' Association website (http://www.ccn-a.co.uk/events/chat-tool) and within e-learning for healthcare under a commons attribution licence.

6. **Do you think it's important to share your failures also, and if so, why?**
It's important for next-generation researchers to hear that the doctoral journey is not always smooth and that there are barriers and forks along the road, but handling these can build transferable skills and resilience as a researcher. For example, we had several unsuccessful funding applications before being awarded funding to deliver the project; however, the feedback enabled us to improve the applications each time. Likewise, submitting papers for publication is not always successful at first attempt and requires rewrites and submission to different journals, which can take time and effort. Life can also throw obstacles in the way. I got divorced at the beginning of my PhD, had a family bereavement and sickness, but my PhD subject, my colleagues, peers and family kept me motivated to complete and succeed. It's important to choose a subject that you are completely passionate about and to have a supportive social network.

7. **Have you ever experienced negativity when it comes to sharing your research successes?**
Finding out that someone else or another team are undertaking a similar study can feel like a negative, but this can sometimes be turned into a positive, as their recommendations can produce further evidence of need for your innovation. Negatives can also include not being successful at first attempt, such as funding applications, submitting papers for publication. They can delay the progress substantially, which is another reason why you need a subject that keeps you motivated to continue.

8. **In your opinion, what is the best way of dealing with negativity?**
Talk to your supervisory team, colleagues, and peers to find out how they manage disappointments. Most researchers will have had similar experiences, and it helps to know that you are not alone.

9. **Now that you have completed your doctorate, do you continue to celebrate your successes and share your failures in the same way or has this changed?**
I have continued to progress my research project since completing my doctorate and celebrate ongoing collaborative achievements through networking, and dissemination via social media, publications, and conferences. I talk about the highs and lows of my doctoral journey with doctoral students, colleagues, and peers, using these experiences to positively shape my doctoral supervisor and PhD course leader role.

10. **What are your top three tips for celebrating and sharing your success in healthcare research?**
    1. Involve patients and the public in your project and share success through public engagement, including with relevant charities and support groups.
    2. Find a professional mentor who has the relevant subject experience and will actively advocate and support you and encourage dissemination of your work.
    3. Evaluate and disseminate the impact of your research.

Professor Kerry Gaskin joined the University of Worcester from Coventry University in 2013 as senior lecturer in children's nursing. She became a principal lecturer in advanced clinical practice in 2016 and an associate professor of nursing in 2022. Her current post is joint with the Three Counties School of Nursing and Midwifery (TCSNM; 2 days/week) and Gloucestershire Hospitals NHSFT (3 days/week). Professor Gaskin is director of studies for three PhD students, course leader for the PhD nursing/midwifery and research and knowledge exchange coordinator for the TCSNM. She is a registered children's nurse and registered adult nurse and worked in children's cardiac intensive care, paediatric intensive care and high dependency care at several specialist children's cardiac units and children's hospitals in the United Kingdom before moving into academia in 2005. Professor Gaskin is the Chairperson of the Congenital Cardiac Nurses Association UK. She completed her PhD in 2017, is a mixed-methods researcher with a particular interest in congenital heart disease, particularly parental home assessment using an early warning tool called the Congenital Heart Assessment Tool (CHAT) to enable parents to identify signs of deterioration in their infants and to make prompt contact with the appropriate health care professional.

CHAPTER 26

Share Your Privilege

Interview with Dr Gita Ramdharry (Neurological Physiotherapy)

1. How did your doctoral research journey begin?

I started my MSc in 2001 and was interested in exploring the effect of orthotics on balance for people with multiple sclerosis. A colleague introduced me to a colleague at UCL, Dr Jonathan Marsden (now a professor at Plymouth University), who was a physiotherapist who had just completed a PhD at the Institute of Neurology. He had an interest in this area and worked as a post-doctoral fellow in the Human Movement Laboratory. I conducted my research in the lab and really loved the environment. Dr Marsden was awarded an MRC clinician scientist fellowship that included funding for a research assistant plus PhD fees. I applied for the job and was fortunately successful, starting my PhD in 2008. It was a pay cut in the short term, but worth it for the learning and where it took my career.

2. During your doctoral experience, did you consider yourself in a position of privilege?

To take on the PhD with a paid wage as part of my job was a huge privilege. Previously I had led a clinical team as a senior physiotherapist, so focussing entirely on my own learning with the PhD process was quite a shift and immensely rewarding. I come from a mixed heritage of Mauritian and Irish parents, so I was the first in my family to have a doctorate. Education is hugely important to many migrant communities, so in a way I was my ancestors' wildest dream (Adonis et al. 2022).

3. How did you seek to pay your experiences forward during the doctoral process?

My first steps on the rung were as a secondary supervisor to PhD students. As I started to acquire my own funding, I looked to support a diverse group of PhD and MRes students. I have supported women with families, navigating their studies part time, and more recently female students from the Middle East and Africa.

4. Why was this important to you?

I know from my own career, the experiences of colleagues and a recent research study I was involved with that there can be a glass ceiling and barriers to progression. I was fortunate to climb to where I am now and I pledged to bring others with me or at least help them to navigate the challenges.

5. What did you learn from your peers, mentors and supervisors in this regard?

For me, the belief in my abilities from mentors and supervisors I respected was really validating and helped me keep my energy and drive. One of my mentors in particular always encouraged me to lean into opportunities when my confidence was at its lowest ebb. My mentors helped me to shape my thinking and showed me where to grow. This also taught me that I needed to share this gift to others.

6. Do you think doctoral students and graduates have a responsibility to share their privilege?

There are many very talented colleagues who just did not have the opportunity to step onto the path that I did. We need to make sure these opportunities are shared and become visible to people who have not been offered these pathways or did not believe they were possible.

7. In your opinion, how should we pay our experiences forward?

Be generous in our offers to provide mentorship. Be open-minded in who we recruit to research roles. Diversity in our teams fosters so much creativity.

8. How do we know if we are paying our experiences forward in the best way?

If your growing team challenges your thinking and makes you work differently, then you know you are getting there. We learn from and with others, so embracing a variety of life experience, cultures and learning styles will ultimately be enriching.

9. Are there any changes or considerations that we need to take on board as part of such a privileged community?

Those of us in more senior positions must put our heads over the parapet to advocate for others. Fight in their corner to widen the opportunities and give them a platform to be heard. Sometimes we need to step to one side and bring new voices through.

10. What are your top three tips for paying it forward?

1. Mentor others to bring them on in their research careers.
2. Get on grant panels and ensure equity, diversity and inclusion are considered with all applicants/applications.
3. Think more openly about who you bring in to work with you on your own research journey.

Dr Gita Ramdharry is a physiotherapist and consultant allied health professional in neuromuscular diseases at the Queen Square/MRC Centre for Neuromuscular Diseases, National Hospital for Neurology and Neurosurgery, UCLH NHS Trust, and an honorary associate professor at UCL.

Gita leads the Neuromuscular Rehabilitation Research Group and is a research supervisor for master's and PhD students, as well as HEE/NIHR ICA clinical doctoral fellows. She has been awarded £930,850 of grant funding as a PI or Co-CI, and £1,741,300 as a co-applicant. Gita has authored 55 articles and 6 book chapters and co-edited 3 books. She is a deputy chair of the HEE/NIHR ICA Clinical Doctoral Academic Fellowships award panels and on scientific panels for Ataxia UK, Myositis UK and CMT UK.

She also works in the area of equality, diversity and inclusion (EDI) and is the chair of the EDI committee for the Department of Neuromuscular Diseases at UCL Institute of Neurology.

Reference

Adonis A, Hammond J, Walumbe J, Wright A, Ramdharry GM. *Disrupting the Status Quo: Global Majority Physiotherapists' Experiences of the Trajectory to Consultant Practice: A Critical Study.* Health Education England; 2022. Available at. https://www.hee.nhs.uk/our-work/allied-health-professions/equality-diversity-inclusion-ahp.

Conclusions

Because when it all come together, it's amazing. When it all comes together, the only thing you can do is bow down in gratitude, as if you have been granted an audience with the divine. Because you have.

—ELIZABETH GILBERT

When you think that your doctorate is all done and dusted and you realise that your research journey is only just beginning, it is exciting and exhilarating to see the potential among the many hills ahead of you.

During my doctorate I often wondered why I did not choose a simpler life. I would look at people in other jobs and think: Why have I chosen this? Why do I always place myself in positions of uncertainty? Why do I always jump into pools where I cannot see the bottom? Soon enough you begin to realise that this is how you learn, and a curious mind is never fulfilled by sitting still or playing safe.

It is in the questioning and in the uncertainty that the good stuff happens. You cannot go over it, under it or around it. You need to and deserve to go through it, finding your way to become a future research leader.

In the end you realise there is no choice: This is who you are, and when you have found your way and the doctoral journey ends, another challenging one will no doubt begin.

Sometimes I have found it difficult to be vulnerable, to reflect and share as openly as I have in this book. However, this is the book I needed to read when I began my journey. I hope that by sharing my way and the ways of other healthcare professionals, it will inspire you to find yours.

Enjoy every moment!

Resources

As a doctoral student, you don't have a lot of time, so here are some extra resources that you may find useful. Although it is not intended to be a prescriptive or exhaustive list, I hope it offers some inspiration.

1. Doctoral studies and writing

Brodzinski E. 2023. *The PhD life raft podcast*. Available at https://thephdliferaft.com/podcast/. Accessed 27 December 2023.

Gilbert E. *Big magic: How to live a creative life, and let go of your fear*. London: Bloomsbury; 2016.

Petre M, Rugg G. *The unwritten rules of PhD research*. 3rd ed. London: McGraw-Hill; 2020.

Phillips EM, Johnson CG. *How to get a PhD: A handbook for students and their supervisors*. 7th ed. Open University Press/McGraw-Hill Education, London; 2022.

Wembury Coaching, 2023. *The PhD life coach podcast*. Available at https://www.thephdlifecoach.com/podcast. Accessed 27 December 2023.

2. Leadership

Brown B. *Dare to lead*. London: Random House Audiobooks; 2018.

Brown B. 2023. *Dare to lead podcast*. Available at https://brenebrown.com/podcast-show/dare-to-lead/. Accessed 16 January 2023.

Cain S. *Quiet: The power of introverts in a world that can't stop talking*. London: Penguin; 2013.

Mohr T. *Playing big: For women who want to speak up, stand out and lead*. 5th ed. Penguin: London; 2022.

3. Productivity

Clear J. *Atomic habits: An easy and proven way to build good habits and break bad ones*. Avery (Penguin): London; 2018.

Covey SR. *The 7 habits of highly effective people: Revised and updated*. 30th ed. Simon and Schuster: London; 2020.

Harvard Business Review. *HBR guide to getting the right work done (HBR guide series)*. Boston, Massachusetts: Harvard Business Review Press; 2013.

Harvard Business Review. *HBR guide to being more productive (HBR guide series)*. Boston, Massachusetts: Harvard Business Review Press; 2017.

4. Well-being

Chatterjee R. *The 4 pillar plan: How to relax, eat, move and sleep your way to a longer, healthier life*. Penguin Life: London; 2018.

Chatterjee R, 2024. *Feel better live more podcast*. Available at https://open.spotify.com/show/6NyPQfcSR9nj0DPDr2ixrK. Accessed 16 January 2024.

Day E. *Failosophy: A handbook for when things go wrong*. (HarperCollins): Glasgow; 2020.

George A, 2024. *Stompcast. The well-being podcast*. Available at https://open.spotify.com/show/5DLl3PO4IklkB9CLRniiGX. Accessed 16 January 2024.

Harvard Business Review. *HBR guide to managing stress at work (HBR guide series)*. Boston, Massachusetts: Harvard Business Review Press; 2014.

INDEX

Note: Page numbers followed by "*f*" indicate figures, "*t*" indicate tables, and "*b*" indicate boxes.